GET IN SHAPE

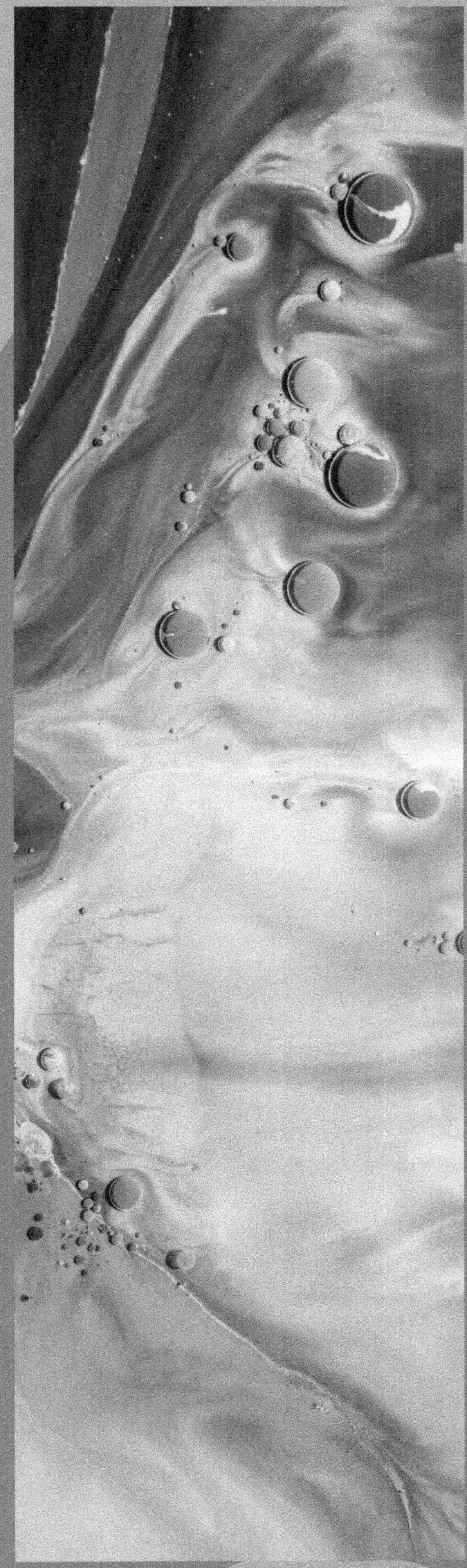

YOU
DESERVE
TO
BE AT
YOUR
BEST
POTENTIAL

LOVE
YOURSELF!
GIVE
YOURSELF
THE BEST!
YOU
DESERVE
IT!

INFO@OFLOWLY.COM

STRENGTH

BE
WHO
YOU
MEANT
TO
BE

R E L A X

THIS BOOK BELONGS TO

____

INFO@OFLOWLY.COM

INTRODUCTION

JOSEPH PILATES, A GERMAN PHYSICAL TRAINER IN THE 20TH CENTURY, DEVELOPED HIS METHOD KNOWN AS 'CONTROLOGY' DURING WORLD WAR I WHILE INTERNED IN A BRITISH CAMP. DRAWING ON HIS BACKGROUND IN YOGA, GYMNASTICS, AND MARTIAL ARTS, PILATES CREATED THIS METHOD TO AID IN THE REHABILITATION OF INJURED SOLDIERS. BY ATTACHING RESISTANCE SPRINGS TO HOSPITAL BEDS, HE DEVISED EXERCISES TO STRENGTHEN MUSCLES AND IMPROVE OVERALL HEALTH AND WELL-BEING.

ONE OF THE GREAT ASPECTS OF PILATES IS ITS ADAPTABILITY TO INDIVIDUAL NEEDS AND ABILITIES. WHETHER RECOVERING FROM INJURY OR SEEKING TO IMPROVE FITNESS, PRACTITIONERS CAN ADJUST THE EXERCISES TO THEIR OWN STRENGTH AND PACE. THIS EMPHASIS ON LISTENING TO ONE'S BODY IS FUNDAMENTAL TO PILATES PRACTICE, ALLOWING PRACTITIONERS TO KNOW WHEN TO PUSH THEMSELVES AND WHEN TO REST.

IN TODAY'S FAST-PACED WORLD, THE IMPORTANCE OF SELF-AWARENESS IS OFTEN OVERLOOKED. PILATES ENCOURAGES A MINDFUL CONNECTION BETWEEN BODY AND MIND, CREATING A DEEPER UNDERSTANDING OF ONESELF AND HOW THE BODY FUNCTIONS. IT'S A VOYAGE OF SELF-DISCOVERY AND EMPOWERMENT, OFFERING INSIGHTS INTO OUR PHYSICAL CAPABILITIES AND LIMITATIONS.

LET'S GO TOGETHER ON THE PILATES JOURNEY THAT WILL GIVE YOU AN ENRICHING EXPERIENCE, ALLOWING INDIVIDUALS LIKE YOU TO UNLOCK YOUR POTENTIAL AND ACHIEVE HOLISTIC WELL-BEING. ISN'T IT AMAZING?

INTRODUCTION

WALL PILATES IS A DIVERSE CREATIVE WAY TO IMPLEMENT TRADITIONAL PILATES EXERCISES INTO A NEW LIFESTYLE. IT BRINGS AN EFFECTIVE, EASY APPROACH TO DEVELOP AND ENHANCE WOMEN'S WELL-BEING AND FITNESS. THIS METHOD USES A WALL AS A RESISTANCE TO PROVIDE THE BEST BENEFITS OF PILATES MOVEMENTS.

WALL PILATES EMPHASIZES ON IMPROVING STRENGTH, FLEXIBILITY, POSTURE, AND OVERALL BODY AWARENESS OF WOMEN WHICH MAKING IT THE PERFECT RECIPE FOR WOMEN OF ALL FITNESS LEVELS AND AGES. EVERYONE CAN GO AT THEIR OWN PACE, RHYTHM AND FLEXIBILITY. IT'S ALL ABOUT LISTENING TO OUR OWN BODY TO GET THE BEST RESULT AND OUTCOME. FORCING MUSCLES IS NOT THE KEY BUT STRETCHING IT AND DOING A CONSISTENT JOB IS.

THE IMPORTANCE OF WALL PILATES IS THE FACT THAT WOMEN NOWADAYS ARE EXTREMELY BUSY. THEY HAVE TO JUGGLE HOUSE CHORES, KIDS, BUSINESSES AND MUCH MORE. IT IS HARD TO FIND A TIME TO RELAX BUT ESPECIALLY HAVING THE FULL PERMISSION TO SET TIME ASIDE FOR THEMSELVES. IN THIS FAST PACED WORLD, WALL PILATES PROVIDES A CONVENIENT, ACCESSIBLE WAY TO STEP INTO HEALTH AND WELLNESS.

IN THE COMFORT OF THEIR OWN HOME, WOMEN CAN DEVELOP AND EXPERIENCE AN IMPROVEMENT ON THEIR STABILITY, ALIGNMENT AND MUSCLES ACTIVATION WHICH PROVIDE AN IMPROVED PHYSICAL CONDITIONING AND INCREASE OF FLEXIBILITY. THOSE POINTS ARE CRUCIAL AS THEY ALLOW YOU TO DECREASE INJURIES IN YOUR DAILY LIFE OR EVEN ACCIDENT AS YOUR BODY GETS STRONGER AND MORE FLEXIBLE. ADDITIONALLY, WALL PILATES OFFERS EMOTIONAL SUPPORT THROUGH STRESS RELIEF, INCREASED ENERGY LEVELS, AND BODY SELF-AWARENESS, HELPING TO MAINTAIN OPTIMAL HEALTH IN TODAY'S BUSY LIFESTYLE.

THE BEAUTY OF THOSE EXERCISES IS ITS SUITABILITY TO WORKOUT FROM YOUR OWN HOME WITH MINIMAL EQUIPMENT REQUIRED. EVEN IF YOU ARE TRAVELING, YOU CAN STILL BE IN SHAPE AND WORK OUT EASILY WITHOUT THE RESTRAINT OF GOING TO THE GYM.IT MAKES IT MORE PROFITABLE AND SUSTAINABLE FOR MODERN LIFESTYLES.

INTRODUCTION

- BOOST INTENSITY: THE WALL PLAYS OUT AS YOUR STRENGTHENING BAND. THE MORE YOU PRESS ON IT THE MORE YOU ADD RESISTANCE TO YOUR MOVEMENTS. IT HELPS TO MAKE IT MORE CHALLENGING AND BUILD STRENGTH AND MUSCLE TONE MORE EFFECTIVELY.

- MUSCLE CONTRACTION: THE BEAUTY OF PUSHING AGAINST THE WALL IS THAT NOT ONLY YOU ARE WORKING YOUR LEGS AND BUTT BUT ALSO YOUR ARMS, CHEST AND SHOULDERS. YOU WILL DISCOVER SOME MUSCLE GROUPS THAT DIDN'T KNOW EXISTED. THE FACT THAT IT IS VERY COMPLETE IT ENGAGES MULTIPLE MUSCLE'S BODY PARTS AND ENHANCES BALANCED MUSCLE DEVELOPMENT.

- STEADINESS AND ALIGNMENT: A STABLE SURFACE IS ESSENTIAL TO PREVENT INJURY. THE WALL SERVES AS THE PERFECT SUPPORT, PROMOTING PROPER BODY ALIGNMENT AND MINIMIZING MISALIGNMENT RISK. THIS SAFE AND EFFECTIVE PRACTICE UTILIZES BODY WEIGHT AND ENHANCES BODY AWARENESS.

- CORE STABILITY: THE IMPORTANCE OF HAVING A WALL AS A RESISTANCE IS THE ACTIVATION GIVEN TO YOUR CORE MUSCLES ALONG WITH YOUR DEEP ABDOMINAL MUSCLE AS WELL AS YOUR BACK MUSCLES. THOSE MUSCLES ARE KEY TO GET A GREAT POSTURE WHERE YOUR PELVIS AND SPINE ARE IN ALIGNMENT. CORE ACTIVATION PROVIDES OPTIMAL POSTURE AND AN OVERALL BODY ALIGNMENT.

- DIVERSITY AND FLEXIBILITY: USING A WALL INTO YOUR PILATES ROUTINE WILL GIVE YOU DIVERSITY AND FLEXIBILITY TO YOUR WORKOUTS. IF YOU WISH, YOU CAN INCORPORATE THE WALL AS YOUR RESISTANCE BAND FOR YOUR TRADITIONAL PILATES EXERCISES. IT WILL GIVE YOU NEW IDEAS AND NEW CHALLENGES ALONG THE WAY.

INTRODUCTION

- CORE STRENGTH: WOMEN RELY ON CORE STRENGTH IN VARIOUS ACTIVITIES, OFTEN WITHOUT REALIZING IT. WALL PILATES SPECIFICALLY TARGETS CORE MUSCLES, INCLUDING THE ABDOMINALS, OBLIQUES, AND LOWER BACK, HELPING WOMEN DEVELOP CORE STRENGTH AND STABILITY. THIS BENEFIT IS KEY FOR IMPROVING POSTURE, REDUCING BACK PAIN, AND ENHANCING OVERALL BODY AWARENESS.

- FLEXIBILITY: WALL PILATES INCLUDES STRETCHING EXERCISES DESIGNED TO ENHANCE FLEXIBILITY AND RANGE OF MOTION. BY INCREASING FLEXIBILITY, WOMEN CAN MOVE MORE FREELY AND COMFORTABLY IN THEIR DAILY ACTIVITIES, WHILE ALSO REDUCING THE RISK OF INJURY.

- STRESS RELIEF: WOMEN OFTEN EXPERIENCE STRESS IN THEIR DAILY LIVES. WALL PILATES OFFERS A BENEFICIAL WAY FOR WOMEN TO RELIEVE STRESS AND TENSION, PROMOTING RELAXATION AND MENTAL WELL-BEING. BY PRACTICING MINDFUL MOVEMENT AND BREATH AWARENESS DURING EXERCISES, WOMEN CAN CULTIVATE A SENSE OF SERENITY AND INNER BALANCE.

BENEFITS FOR SENIOR WOMEN:

- FALL PREVENTION: THE FLAT SURFACE OF THE WALL PROVIDES STABLE AND SECURE SUPPORT, ENABLING SENIOR WOMEN TO EXERCISE EFFECTIVELY WITHOUT THE RISK OF INJURY. THIS OPTION IS INVALUABLE FOR SENIOR WOMEN AS IT SIGNIFICANTLY REDUCES THE RISK OF FALLS AND INJURIES ASSOCIATED WITH BALANCE PROBLEMS.

- JOINT HEALTH: WALL PILATES EXERCISES ARE DESIGNED TO BE GENTLE ON THE JOINTS WHILE STILL DELIVERING A CHALLENGING WORKOUT, MAKING THEM IDEAL FOR SENIORS WITH ARTHRITIS OR JOINT PAIN.

- IMPROVED MOBILITY: REGULAR PRACTICE OF WALL PILATES CAN ENHANCE MOBILITY AND RANGE OF MOTION IN SENIOR WOMEN, ENABLING THEM TO MAINTAIN INDEPENDENCE AND PERFORM DAILY ACTIVITIES WITH EASE.

INTRODUCTION

BENEFITS FOR INDIVIDUALS OF ALL LEVELS:

- STRENGTH: WALL PILATES HELPS INDIVIDUALS BUILD STRENGTH AND MUSCLE TONE THROUGHOUT THE BODY, INCLUDING THE CORE, ARMS, LEGS, AND BACK.

- FOCUSED ON BALANCE AND COORDINATION: WALL PILATES OFFER AN INCREASE OF BALANCE AND STABILITY EXERCISES, IMPROVING COORDINATION WHICH HELPS TO REDUCE RISK OF FALLS AND ENHANCES OVERALL ATHLETICISM.

- MIND-BODY CONNECTION: WALL PILATES EMPHASIZES MINDFULNESS AND BODY AWARENESS, HELPING INDIVIDUALS CONNECT WITH THEIR BODIES ON A DEEPER LEVEL AND IMPROVE THEIR OVERALL WELL-BEING.

NOW, IT'S YOUR TURN.
GET READY TO ACHIEVE YOUR DESIRED GOALS WITH THIS WONDERFUL TECHNIQUE.

THERE'S NO NEED TO PURCHASE ANY EQUIPMENT – YOU CAN START RIGHT AWAY. NO MORE EXCUSES, NO MORE WAITING.
YOUR TIME IS NOW.

I'M EXCITED TO EMBARK ON THIS JOURNEY WITH YOU THROUGH THE PAGES, AND I CAN'T WAIT TO SEE THE LOOK ON YOUR FACE WHEN YOU REALIZE YOU'RE GETTING STRONGER, MORE FLEXIBLE, AND STABLE.

LET'S MAKE IT HAPPEN TOGETHER!

INTRODUCTION

LEVERAGING THE POWER OF OUR MINDS AND IMAGINATION IS TRULY TRANSFORMATIVE. IT'S REMARKABLE HOW OUR THOUGHTS CAN SHAPE OUR REALITY AND INFLUENCE OUR OUTCOMES. LET ME SHARE MY PERSPECTIVE ON THIS IN A MORE PERSONAL AND UNIQUE WAY:

IMAGINE THIS: BEFORE YOU EVEN BEGIN YOUR WORKOUT, CLOSE YOUR EYES AND VISUALIZE YOURSELF PERFORMING EACH EXERCISE WITH PRECISION AND GRACE. FEEL THE MUSCLES ENGAGING, THE BREATH FLOWING SMOOTHLY, AND THE BODY MOVING WITH PURPOSE. AS YOU IMMERSE YOURSELF IN THIS MENTAL REHEARSAL, YOU'RE NOT JUST ENVISIONING THE MOVEMENTS – YOU'RE SENDING POWERFUL SIGNALS TO YOUR BRAIN, PRIMING IT FOR ACTION AND IGNITING A SENSE OF READINESS WITHIN.

IT'S LIKE SETTING THE STAGE FOR SUCCESS BEFORE EVEN STEPPING ONTO IT. BY VISUALIZING YOUR DESIRED OUTCOMES AND EMBODYING THE SENSATION OF ACHIEVEMENT, YOU'RE ALIGNING YOUR MIND AND BODY IN PERFECT HARMONY. AND THE BEAUTY OF IT ALL?

THIS MENTAL PREPARATION DOESN'T JUST ENHANCE YOUR PERFORMANCE – IT CAN ALSO BRING A PROFOUND SENSE OF PEACE AND FOCUS TO YOUR WORKOUT SESSIONS.

BUT IT DOESN'T STOP THERE.

INTRODUCTION

VISUALIZING THE IMPACT OF EACH EXERCISE ON YOUR BODY TAKES IT TO A WHOLE NEW LEVEL.

PICTURE YOUR MUSCLES TONING AND STRENGTHENING WITH EVERY REP, ENVISIONING YOURSELF BECOMING LEANER, STRONGER, AND MORE VIBRANT WITH EACH MOVEMENT. IT'S A HOLISTIC APPROACH TO FITNESS THAT GOES BEYOND THE PHYSICAL REALM, TAPPING INTO THE POWER OF YOUR IMAGINATION TO AMPLIFY YOUR RESULTS.

NOW, I KNOW IT MIGHT SOUND A BIT UNCONVENTIONAL, EVEN CONTROVERSIAL TO SOME. BUT LET ME TELL YOU, I'VE EXPERIENCED FIRSTHAND THE INCREDIBLE EFFECTS OF VISUALIZATION IN MY OWN FITNESS JOURNEY.

TIME AND TIME AGAIN, I'VE WITNESSED HOW ENVISIONING MY GOALS AND OUTCOMES DURING EXERCISE HAS ACCELERATED MY PROGRESS AND PROPELLED ME TOWARDS SUCCESS.

OF COURSE, IT'S IMPORTANT TO PAIR THIS MENTAL PRACTICE WITH PROPER TECHNIQUE AND A BALANCED DIET – THAT'S NON-NEGOTIABLE. BUT BY TAPPING INTO THE LIMITLESS POTENTIAL OF YOUR IMAGINATION, YOU CAN SUPERCHARGE YOUR EFFORTS AND UNLOCK NEW LEVELS OF ACHIEVEMENT.

SO WHY NOT GIVE IT A TRY? YOU'VE GOT NOTHING TO LOSE AND EVERYTHING TO GAIN. EMBRACE THE POWER OF VISUALIZATION, AND WATCH AS YOUR FITNESS JOURNEY TAKES ON A WHOLE NEW DIMENSION OF POSSIBILITY.

INTRODUCTION

IT'S A BIT OF A DIFFERENT BALL GAME COMPARED TO OTHER FITNESS TECHNIQUES. PATIENCE IS THE NAME OF THE GAME HERE. UNLIKE THOSE QUICK-FIX WORKOUTS PROMISING INSTANT RESULTS, WALL PILATES REQUIRES TIME AND DEDICATION.

WE ALL KNOW THAT THERE ARE NO QUICK FIXES IN LIFE. WE LIVE IN A FAST FOOD, IMMEDIATE SOCIETY THAT HAS A HARD TIME TO WAIT AND BE PATIENT FOR THINGS. NONETHELESS, YOU WILL SEE INCREDIBLE LASTING RESULTS IF YOU DO.

THOSE CHISELED ABS OR SCULPTED MUSCLES WON'T BE SEEN OVERNIGHT. IT TAKES AT LEAST A MONTH OF CONSISTENT PRACTICE BEFORE YOU START NOTICING SOME REAL DEFINITION AND PROGRESS. BUT LET ME TELL YOU, WHEN THOSE CHANGES START APPEARING, IT'S LIKE UNCOVERING HIDDEN TREASURES – UNEXPECTED AND OH-SO-SATISFYING.

NOW, HERE'S THE THING – WALL PILATES ISN'T JUST ABOUT THE PHYSICAL GRIND. IT'S ABOUT FORGING A DEEP CONNECTION BETWEEN YOUR BODY AND MIND. IT'S ABOUT LEARNING TO LISTEN TO THE SUBTLE WHISPERS OF YOUR BODY AND UNDERSTANDING HOW IT FUNCTIONS.
AND TRUST ME, THE REWARDS GO FAR BEYOND TONED MUSCLES AND IMPROVED FLEXIBILITY. YOU'LL FIND YOURSELF FEELING MORE CENTERED, MORE GROUNDED, WITH EACH SESSION.

AND WHEN THE GOING GETS TOUGH, THOSE MINDFUL BREATHS WILL BE YOUR ANCHOR, GUIDING YOU BACK TO A PLACE OF CALM AND CLARITY.

BUT HERE'S WHERE THE MAGIC TRULY LIES – WITH WALL PILATES, YOU'RE NOT JUST STRENGTHENING YOUR OUTER SHELL; YOU'RE NOURISHING YOUR INNER BEING TOO.

IT'S A HOLISTIC JOURNEY OF SELF-DISCOVERY AND SELF-IMPROVEMENT, WHERE EVERY MOVEMENT IS A STEP CLOSER TO ALIGNING YOUR BODY, MIND, AND SOUL.

AND THE BEST PART? YOU CAN EMBARK ON THIS TRANSFORMATIVE JOURNEY RIGHT IN THE COMFORT OF YOUR OWN HOME.

INTRODUCTION

TIPS BEFORE GETTING STARTED:

BEFORE THE WALL PILATES EXERCISES:

STARTING YOUR WALL PILATES WITH A LIGHT CARDIO SUCH AS A WALK, A JOGGING IN PLACE FOLLOWED BY SOME STRETCHES WILL PREPARE YOUR BODY TO GET READY.

WHILE EXERCISING:

- ENGAGE YOUR VISUALIZATION, ENGAGE YOUR CORE AND SPINE AT ALL TIME.
- START SLOW AND LISTEN TO YOUR BODY. GO AT YOUR OWN PACE. YOU WILL GET THE BEST RESULTS. EXERCISING IS NOT ABOUT BEING BRUTAL WITH OURSELVES BUT GIVING THE RIGHT AMOUNT OF PUSH AND PRESSURE THAT YOUR BODY NEEDS. YOU ARE THE BEST TO KNOW WHAT IT NEEDS.
- BREATHE DEEPLY BEFORE, DURING AND AFTER EACH EXERCISES. DON'T HOLD YOUR BREATHE AS IT COULD CREATE TENSIONS IN YOUR BODY.
- DON'T FORGET TO DRINK WATER AND STAY HYDRATED AS IT'S KEY TO MAINTAIN YOUR ENERGY LEVELS. BUT ALSO WILL HELP YOUR MUSCLES TO GIVE YOU AN OPTIMAL PERFORMANCE.

AFTER EXERCISING:

HAVING A COOL DOWN OF A FEW STRETCHES WILL LOWER YOUR HEART RATE AND WILL BRING FLEXIBILITY TO YOUR OWN BODY.

INTRODUCTION

WELCOME TO A JOURNEY UNLIKE ANY OTHER – A JOURNEY GOING THROUGH REALMS OF MOTIVATION AND SELF-DISCOVERY.

THIS BOOK ISN'T JUST ABOUT WORKING OUT; IT'S ABOUT IGNITING THE FIRE WITHIN YOU, EMPOWERING YOU TO EMBRACE EACH EXERCISE WITH PURPOSE AND PASSION.

AS YOU FLIP THROUGH THESE PAGES, YOU'LL FIND MORE THAN JUST COLORFUL PICTURES AND WORKOUT ROUTINES. YOU'LL DISCOVER A TREASURE TROVE OF MOTIVATIONAL PHRASES, CAREFULLY CURATED TO INSPIRE AND UPLIFT YOU ON YOUR 28-DAY JOURNEY.

EACH PHRASE IS LIKE A GENTLE WHISPER OF ENCOURAGEMENT, URGING YOU TO PUSH BEYOND YOUR LIMITS AND EMBRACE YOUR FULL POTENTIAL.

BUT THIS BOOK ISN'T JUST ABOUT SCULPTING YOUR BODY – IT'S ABOUT NOURISHING YOUR SOUL. IT'S ABOUT ALIGNING YOUR BODY, MIND, AND SPIRIT TO CREATE A HARMONIOUS SYMPHONY OF WELLNESS WHICH IS SELF-LOVE, RESPECT, AND GRACE TO UNLOCKING WHO YOU ARE FULLY MEANT TO BE.

SO, TAKE MY HAND AND LET'S GO TOGETHER ON THIS ADVENTURE; SWEAT, STRETCH, AND GROW – NOT JUST PHYSICALLY, BUT EMOTIONALLY AND SPIRITUALLY AS WELL. TOGETHER, WE'LL WEAVE A TAPESTRY OF STRENGTH, RESILIENCE, AND JOY THAT WILL CARRY US THROUGH LIFE'S UPS AND DOWNS.

ARE YOU READY TO EXPLORE THE DEPTHS OF YOUR POTENTIAL? YOU CAN DO IT.

YOUR BODY AWAITS FOR THIS MOMENT TO CONNECT WITH YOU EVEN MORE DEEPLY.

MOTIVATIONS:

PART 1

GET READY FOR YOUR 28 DAY CHALLENGE :

IT MAY SEEM TOO EASY BUT REPETITION IS KEY. YOU'LL FEEL IT!

DAY 1-4: LAYING FOUNDATION

WARM UP:	PICK 2 EXERCISES FROM PAGE 17-21
WALL SQUATS: 3 SETS OF 10 REPS	PAGE 22
SINGLE LEG GLUTE BRIDGE: 3 SETS OF 12 REPS ON EACH LEG	PAGE 23
CRUNCHES: 3 SETS OF 12 REPS	PAGE 24
TOE TAP CRUNCH: 3 SETS OF 12 REPS	PAGE 26
WALL PUSH-UPS: 3 SETS OF 10 REPS	PAGE 25
FROG CRUNCHES: 3 SETS OF 12 REPS	PAGE 27
COOL DOWN	PICK 2 EXERCISES FROM PAGE 47-51

DAY 5-9: BUILDING ON

WARM UP:	PICK 2 EXERCISES FROM PAGE 17-21
SIDE PLANK HIP OPENER - RIGHT/LEFT: HOLD FOR 30 SECONDS, THEN PERFORM 10 HIP OPENERS ON EACH SIDE	PAGE 29
HALF MOON LEG LIFTS - RIGHT/LEFT: PERFORM 3 SETS OF 10 REPS ON EACH SIDE	PAGE P46
FROG CRUNCHES: 3 SETS OF 12 REPS	PAGE 27
RAINBOWS: 3 SETS OF 12 REPS	PAGE 31
COOL DOWN	PICK 2 EXERCISES FROM PAGE 47-51

'YOU ARE SO LOVABLE.'

GET READY FOR YOUR 28 DAY CHALLENGE :

PART 2

DAY 10-14: INTERMEDIATE

WARM UP:	PICK 2 EXERCISES FROM PAGE 17-21
WALL SQUAT WITH LEG LIFTS: 3 SETS OF 10 REPS ON EACH LEG	PAGE 28
HIP OPENER TO LEG EXTEND - RIGHT/LEFT: 3 SETS OF 10 REPS ON EACH SIDE	PAGE 30
WALL PLANK WITH SHOULDER TAPS: HOLD FOR 30 SECONDS, ALTERNATE TAPPING SHOULDERS FOR 10 REPS	PAGE 32
WALL BRIDGE WITH MARCHING: 3 SETS OF 12 REPS	PAGE 33
RAINBOWS: 3 SETS OF 15 REPS	PAGE 31
COOL DOWN:	PICK 2 EXERCISES FROM PAGE 47-51

DAY 15-19: GETTING STRONGER

WARM UP:	PICK 2 EXERCISES FROM PAGE 17-21
WALL PLANK WITH SHOULDER TAPS: HOLD FOR 30 SECONDS, ALTERNATE TAPPING SHOULDERS FOR 12 REPS	PAGE 32
JUMPING WALL SQUATS: 3 SETS OF 10 REPS	PAGE 34
WALL BRIDGE WITH ALTERNATING LEG EXTENSIONS: 3 SETS OF 12 REPS	PAGE 37
FIRE HYDRANT TO BUTT PULSE - RIGHT/LEFT: 3 SETS OF 10 REPS	PAGE 45
CRUNCHES: 3 SETS OF 12 REPS	PAGE 24
COOL DOWN:	PICK 2 EXERCISES FROM PAGE 47-51

"YOU ARE GETTING STRONGER."

GET READY FOR YOUR
28 DAY CHALLENGE :

DAY 20-24: POWER/ENDURANCE

WARM UP:	PICK 2 EXERCISES FROM PAGE 17-21
EXPLOSIVE WALL PUSH-UPS: 3 SETS OF 8 REPS	PAGE 35
WALL PLANK WITH KNEE DRIVES: HOLD FOR 30 SECONDS, BRING EACH KNEE TOWARDS CHEST FOR 10 REPS	PAGE 36
WALL BRIDGE WITH ALTERNATING LEG EXTENSIONS: 3 SETS OF 12 REPS EACH SIDE	PAGE 37
WALL PIKE PRESS: 3 SETS OF 8 REPS	PAGE 38
SIDE PLANK HIP OPENER – RIGHT/LEFT: HOLD FOR 30 SECONDS, THEN 10 HIP OPENERS ON EACH SIDE	PAGE 29
COOL DOWN	PAGE 48-49

DAY 25-28: END GOAL

WARM UP:	PICK 2 EXERCISES FROM PAGE 17-21
WALL SQUAT TO BUTTERFLY CRUNCH: 3 SETS OF 10 REPS	PAGE 39
SINGLE LEG GLUTE BRIDGE TO TOE TAP CRUNCH: 3 SETS OF 12 REPS ON EACH LEG	PAGE 40
CRUNCHES TO FROG CRUNCHES SUPERSET: 3 SETS OF 15 REPS FOR EACH EXERCISE	PAGE 41
TOE TAP CRUNCH TO HIP OPENER TO LEG EXTEND – RIGHT SUPERSET: 3 SETS OF 12 REPS FOR EACH EXERCISE	PAGE 43
FROG CRUNCHES TO RAINBOWS SUPERSET: 3 SETS OF 12 REPS FOR EACH EXERCISE	PAGE 44
COOL DOWN	PAGE 47-48

'YOU ARE AN ACHIEVER."

WARM UP:

1. LEG SWING RIGHT AND LEFT: 10 X EACH SIDE

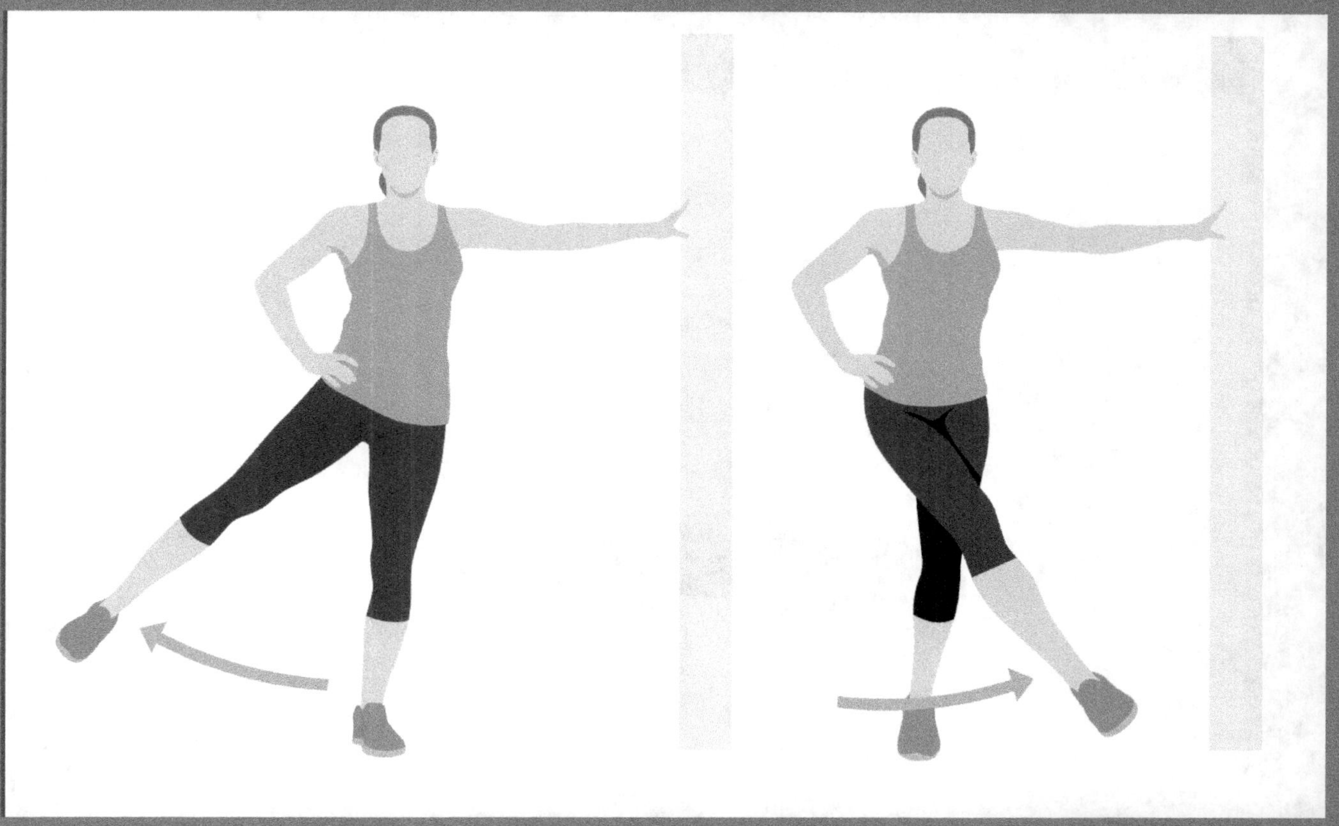

1. STAND UPRIGHT WITH YOUR FEET HIP-WIDTH APART AND YOUR ARMS RELAXED BY YOUR SIDES.
2. ENGAGE YOUR CORE MUSCLES TO STABILIZE YOUR TORSO AND MAINTAIN GOOD POSTURE THROUGHOUT THE EXERCISE.
3. SHIFT YOUR WEIGHT ONTO YOUR RIGHT LEG AND SLIGHTLY BEND YOUR RIGHT KNEE.
4. KEEPING YOUR LEFT LEG STRAIGHT, BEGIN TO SWING IT FORWARD AND BACKWARD IN A CONTROLLED MOTION.
5. THEN, SWING YOUR LEFT LEG BACKWARD, EXTENDING IT BEHIND YOU WHILE KEEPING IT STRAIGHT.
6. AS YOU SWING YOUR LEGS, FOCUS ON MAINTAINING A STABLE PELVIS AND AVOIDING EXCESSIVE MOVEMENT IN YOUR UPPER BODY.
7. KEEP YOUR MOVEMENTS SMOOTH AND CONTROLLED, AVOIDING ANY JERKING OR SWINGING OF THE TORSO.

BENEFITS: HELPS IMPROVE YOUR HIP FLEXIBILITY, RANGE OF MOTION, AND OVERALL LOWER BODY FUNCTION,

WARM UP:

2. PLIÉ PULSES 10 X

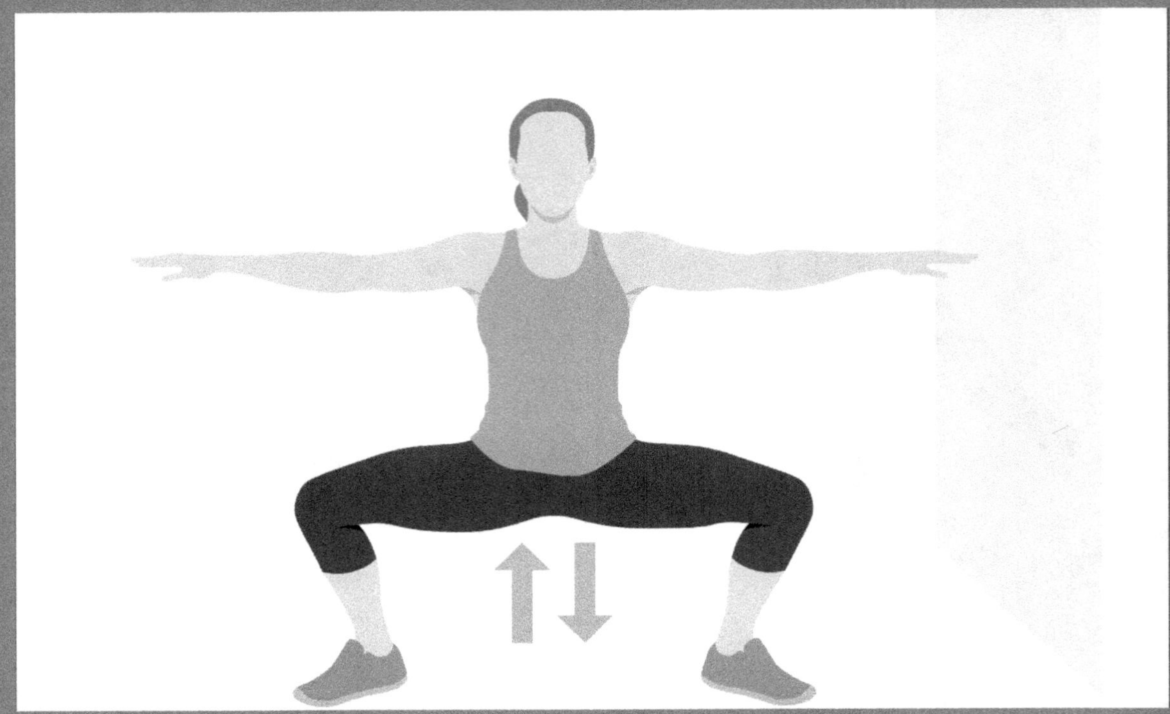

1. BEND YOUR KNEES AND LOWER YOUR BODY INTO A SQUAT POSITION, KEEPING YOUR BACK STRAIGHT AND YOUR WEIGHT IN YOUR HEELS.
2. ONCE YOU REACH THE LOWEST POINT OF YOUR SQUAT WHERE YOUR THIGHS ARE PARALLEL TO THE FLOOR (OR AS LOW AS COMFORTABLE), HOLD THIS POSITION.
3. FROM THE SQUAT POSITION, BEGIN TO PULSE UP AND DOWN IN A SMALL RANGE OF MOTION, MOVING ONLY A FEW INCHES UP AND DOWN.
4. FOCUS ON CONTRACTING YOUR LEG MUSCLES WITH EACH PULSE, KEEPING TENSION IN YOUR THIGHS AND GLUTES.
5. KEEP YOUR BREATHING STEADY AND RHYTHMICAL, EXHALING AS YOU PULSE UP AND INHALING AS YOU LOWER DOWN.

BENEFITS; HELPS STRENGTHEN AND TONE THE MUSCLES OF THE LEGS AND GLUTES.

3. HIP ROTATION   10 X EACH SIDE

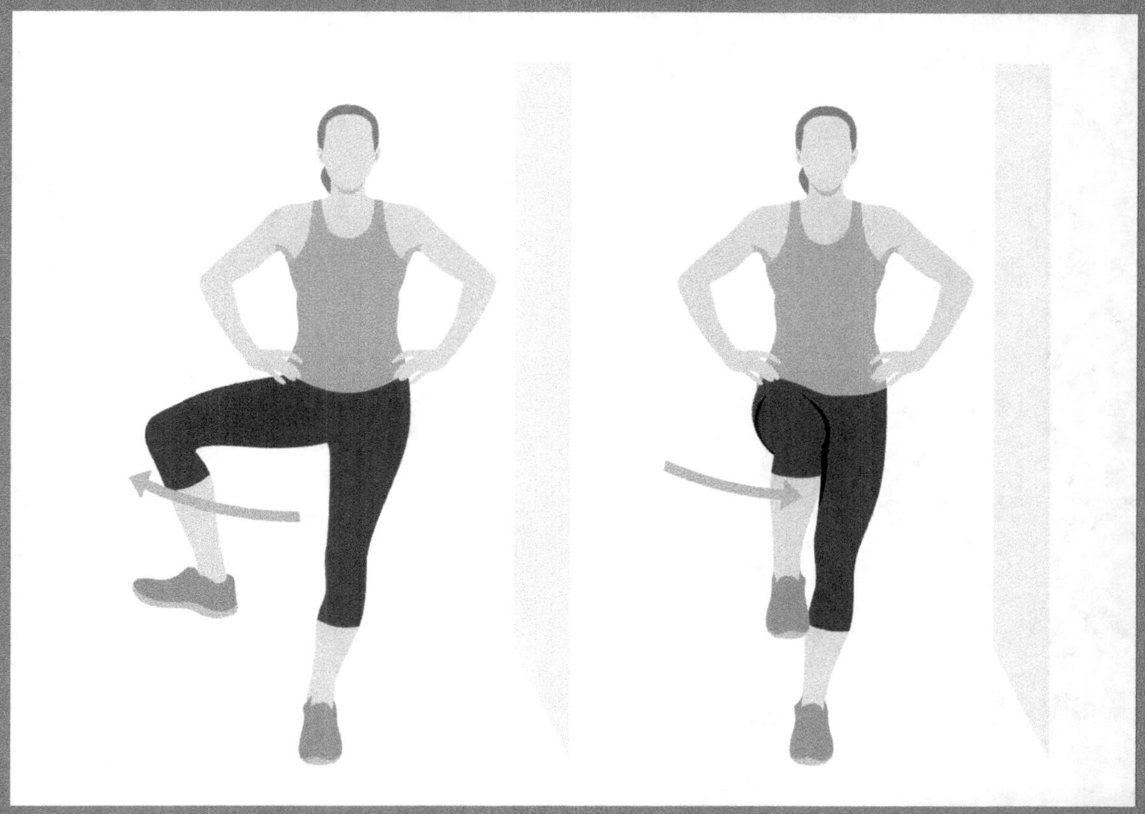

1. BEGIN BY SHIFTING YOUR WEIGHT ONTO YOUR RIGHT LEG WHILE KEEPING YOUR LEFT LEG RELAXED.
2. SLOWLY ROTATE YOUR LEFT HIP OUTWARD, AWAY FROM YOUR BODY, AS FAR AS COMFORTABLE WITHOUT FORCING THE MOVEMENT.
3. HOLD THE END POSITION FOR A MOMENT, FEELING A GENTLE STRETCH IN THE HIP AND GROIN AREA.
4. RETURN YOUR LEFT HIP TO THE STARTING POSITION, BRINGING IT BACK TO NEUTRAL.
5. REPEAT THE ROTATION MOVEMENT ON THE LEFT SIDE, SHIFTING YOUR WEIGHT ONTO YOUR LEFT LEG AND ROTATING YOUR RIGHT HIP OUTWARD.
6. CONTINUE ALTERNATING HIP ROTATIONS FROM SIDE TO SIDE IN A CONTROLLED MANNER, FOCUSING ON SMOOTH AND FLUID MOVEMENTS.

BENEFITS: HELPS TO ALLEVIATE STIFFNESS AND TIGHTNESS IN THE HIPS. HELPS LUBRICATING THE JOINT AND INCREASING BLOOD FLOW TO THE SURROUNDING MUSCLES AND TISSUES.

'YOU HAVE A WELL INSIDE OF YOU."

WARM UP:

4. WALL ROLL DOWN 10 X

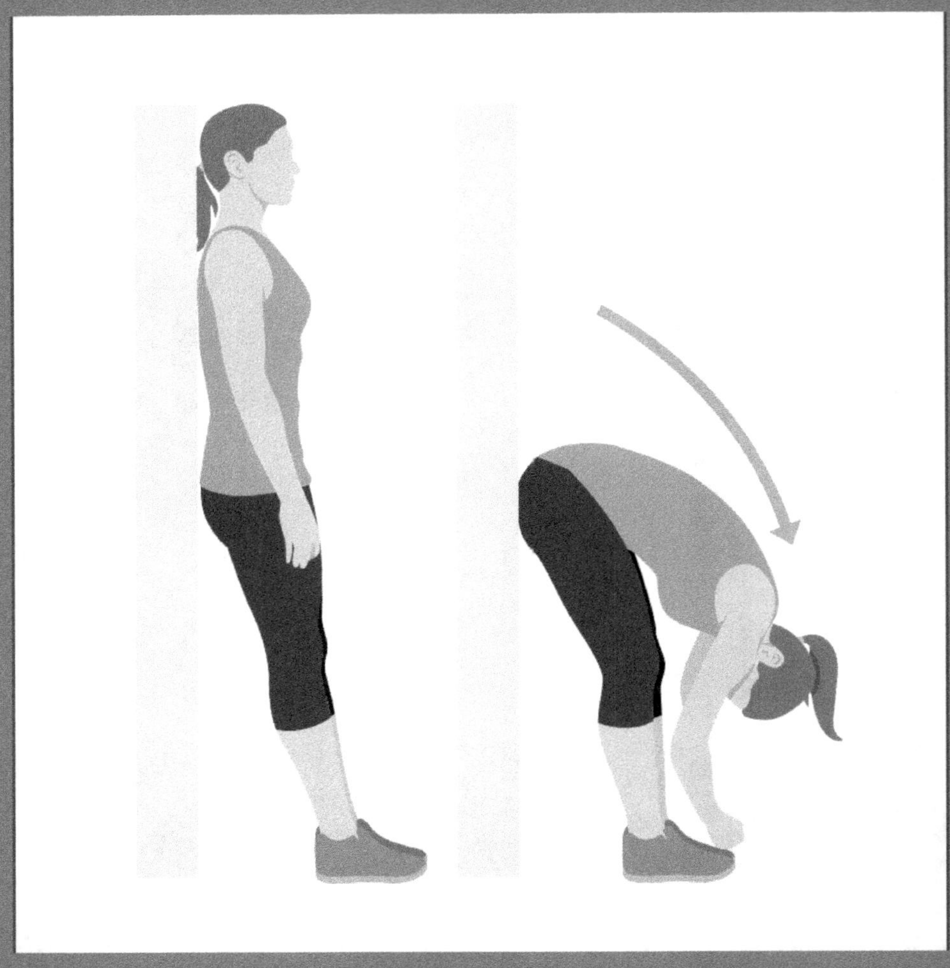

1. STAND WITH YOUR BACK AGAINST A WALL.
2. SLOWLY EXHALE AS YOU SEQUENTIALLY ROLL YOUR SPINE DOWN.
3. REACH TOWARDS THE FLOOR. HOLD THE STRETCH BRIEFLY.
4. THEN ENGAGE YOUR CORE TO ROLL BACK UP TO STANDING.

BENEFITS: HELPS WITH STRESS RELIEF AND RELAXATION.

WARM UP:

5. TORSO ROTATION 10 X

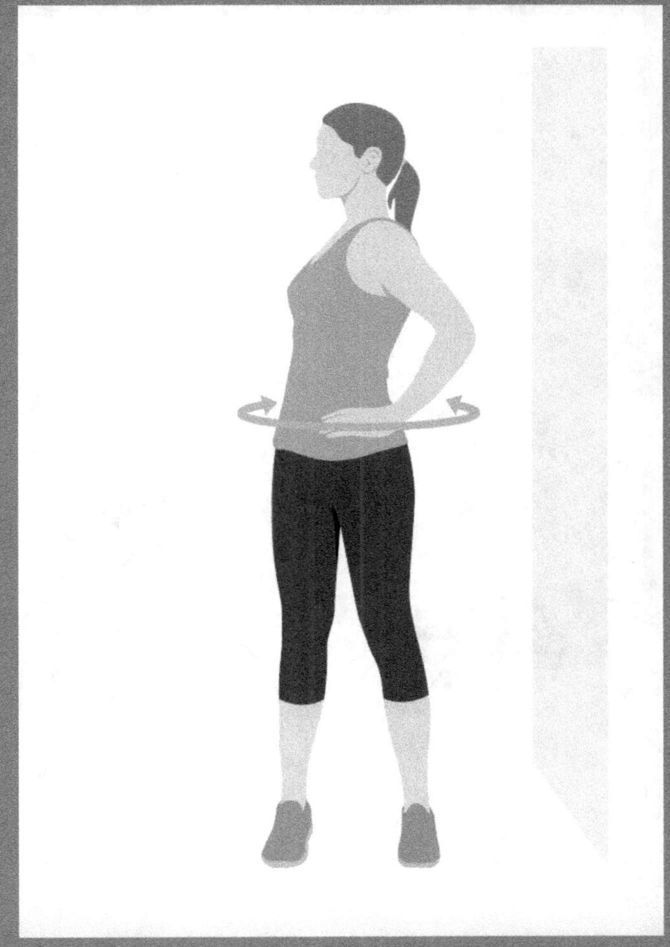

1. STAND TALL WITH YOUR FEET SHOULDER-WIDTH APART AND YOUR KNEES SLIGHTLY BENT. KEEP YOUR ARMS RELAXED BY YOUR SIDES.
2. TIGHTEN YOUR ABDOMINAL MUSCLES TO STABILIZE YOUR TORSO.
3. SLOWLY TWIST YOUR UPPER BODY TO ONE SIDE, KEEPING YOUR HIPS FACING FORWARD. ALLOW YOUR ARMS TO SWING NATURALLY WITH THE MOVEMENT.
4. HOLD THE TWIST BRIEFLY, FEELING THE STRETCH IN YOUR SIDES. THEN, SLOWLY RETURN TO THE STARTING POSITION.
5. REPEAT ON THE OTHER SIDE: TWIST YOUR TORSO TO THE OPPOSITE SIDE, AGAIN HOLDING BRIEFLY BEFORE RETURNING TO THE CENTER.

BENEFITS: HELPS IMPROVE CORE STRENGTH AND FLEXIBILITY, AS WELL AS MOBILITY IN THE SPINE.

"DON'T LET YOUR MINDSET STOP YOU. KEEP VISUALIZING IT."

28 DAY CHALLENGE:

1. WALL SQUATS

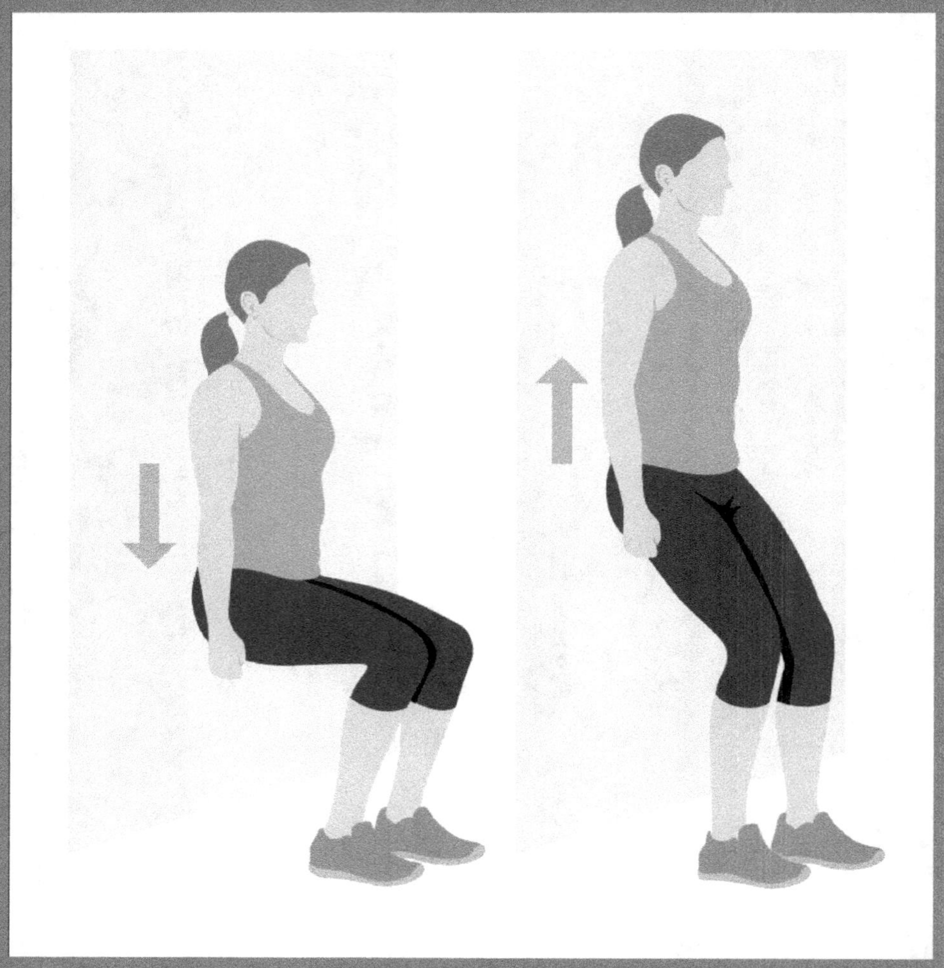

1. STAND WITH YOUR BACK AGAINST A WALL AND YOUR FEET HIP-WIDTH APART, ABOUT 1-2 FEET AWAY FROM THE WALL.
2. SLOWLY SLIDE DOWN THE WALL BY BENDING YOUR KNEES, AS IF SITTING INTO A CHAIR. KEEP YOUR BACK AGAINST THE WALL AND YOUR KNEES ALIGNED WITH YOUR ANKLES.
3. ENSURE YOUR KNEES STAY DIRECTLY ABOVE YOUR ANKLES AND DON'T EXTEND PAST YOUR TOES. KEEP YOUR SPINE STRAIGHT AND ENGAGE YOUR CORE MUSCLES.
4. HOLD THE SQUAT POSITION FOR A FEW SECONDS, FOCUSING ON KEEPING YOUR WEIGHT IN YOUR HEELS AND YOUR THIGHS PARALLEL TO THE FLOOR.
5. PUSH THROUGH YOUR HEELS TO STRAIGHTEN YOUR LEGS AND RETURN TO THE STARTING POSITION.

BENEFITS: HELPS STRENGTHEN THE MUSCLES OF THE LOWER BODY, INCLUDING THE QUADRICEPS, HAMSTRINGS, AND GLUTES, WHILE ALSO IMPROVING STABILITY AND ENDURANCE.

28 DAY CHALLENGE:

2.

SINGLE LEG GLUTE BRIDGE

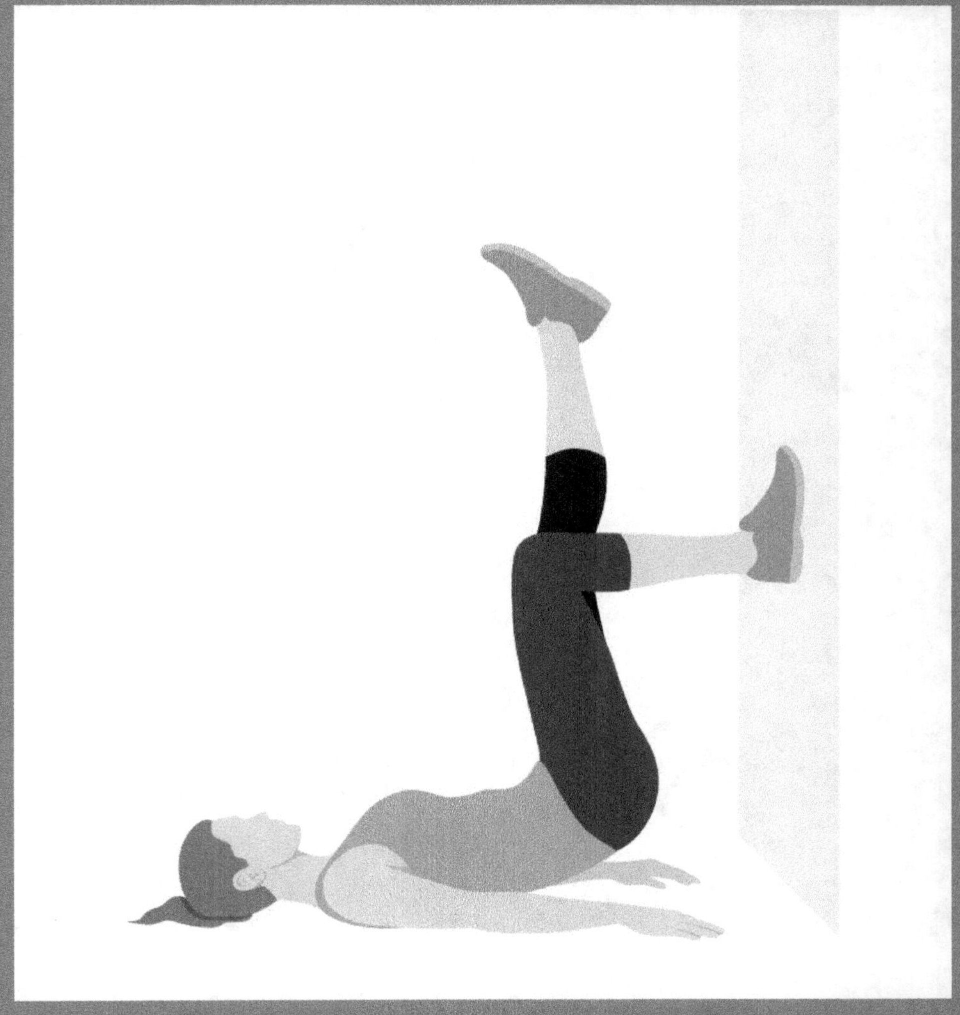

1. LIE ON YOUR BACK WITH YOUR FEET FLAT AGAINST A WALL, KNEES BENT, AND ARMS BY YOUR SIDES.
2. EXTEND ONE LEG STRAIGHT UP TOWARDS THE CEILING, PRESSING YOUR FOOT AGAINST THE WALL.
3. DRAW YOUR NAVEL TOWARDS YOUR SPINE TO ENGAGE YOUR CORE MUSCLES.
4. EXHALE AS YOU PRESS THROUGH THE FOOT ON THE WALL, LIFTING YOUR HIPS TOWARDS THE CEILING, FORMING A STRAIGHT LINE FROM SHOULDERS TO KNEES.
5. AT THE TOP OF THE MOVEMENT, SQUEEZE YOUR GLUTES TO MAXIMIZE ENGAGEMENT.
6. INHALE AS YOU SLOWLY LOWER YOUR HIPS BACK DOWN TOWARDS THE MAT WITHOUT TOUCHING THE GROUND.

BENEFITS: HELPS TARGETS THE GLUTES, HAMSTRINGS, AND CORE MUSCLES, PROMOTING LOWER BODY STRENGTH AND STABILITY.

"YOUR BODY LOVES YOU."

28 DAY CHALLENGE:

3.   CRUNCHES

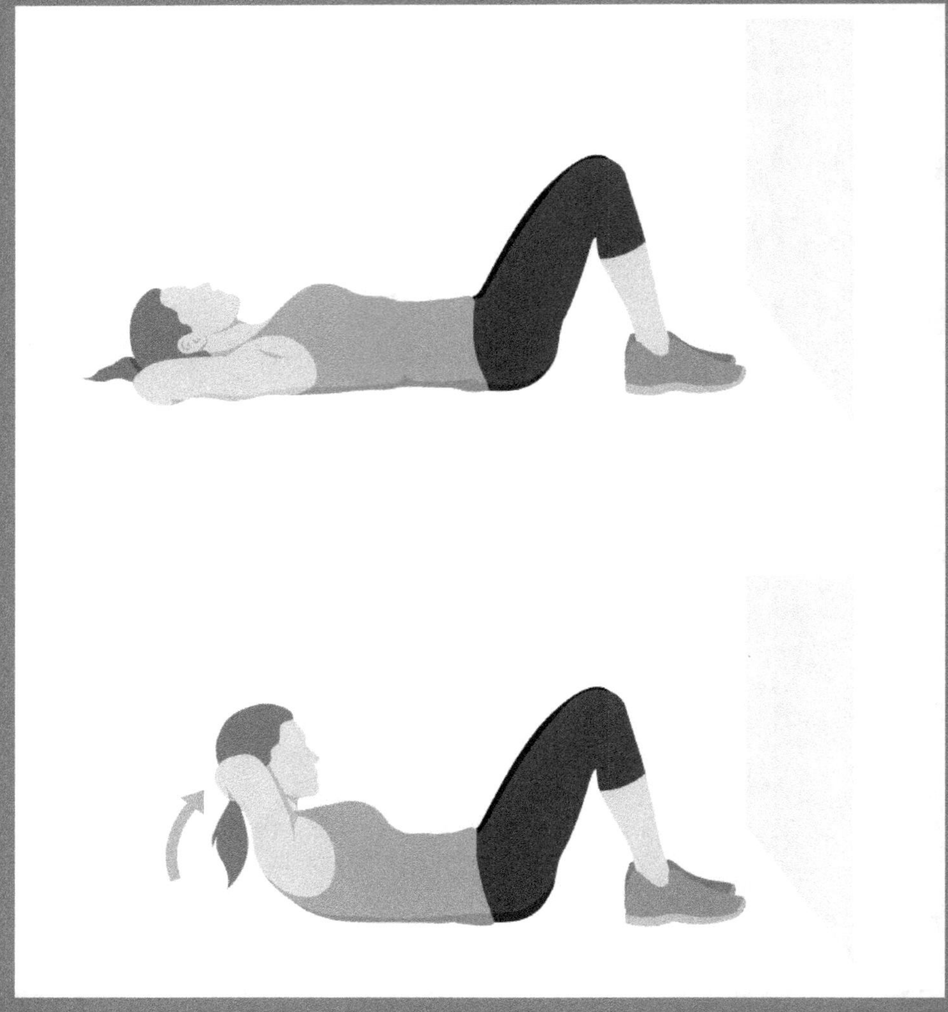

1. LIE ON YOUR BACK WITH YOUR FEET FLAT AGAINST A WALL AND YOUR KNEES BENT AT A 90-DEGREE ANGLE. KEEP YOUR ARMS BY YOUR SIDES OR CROSSED OVER YOUR CHEST.
2. DRAW YOUR NAVEL (BELLY BUTTON) TOWARDS YOUR SPINE TO ENGAGE YOUR ABDOMINAL MUSCLES.
3. EXHALE AS YOU LIFT YOUR HEAD, NECK, AND SHOULDERS OFF THE MAT, AIMING TO BRING YOUR RIBCAGE TOWARDS YOUR HIPS.
4. HOLD THE CRUNCH POSITION BRIEFLY, MAINTAINING TENSION IN YOUR ABDOMINAL MUSCLES.
5. INHALE AS YOU SLOWLY LOWER YOUR UPPER BODY BACK TOWARDS THE MAT, KEEPING CONTROL OF THE MOVEMENT.

BENEFITS: HELPS ENGAGE THE ABDOMINAL MUSCLES EFFECTIVELY WHILE PROVIDING SUPPORT FOR THE LOWER BACK.

28 DAY CHALLENGE:

4.   WALL PUSH-UPS

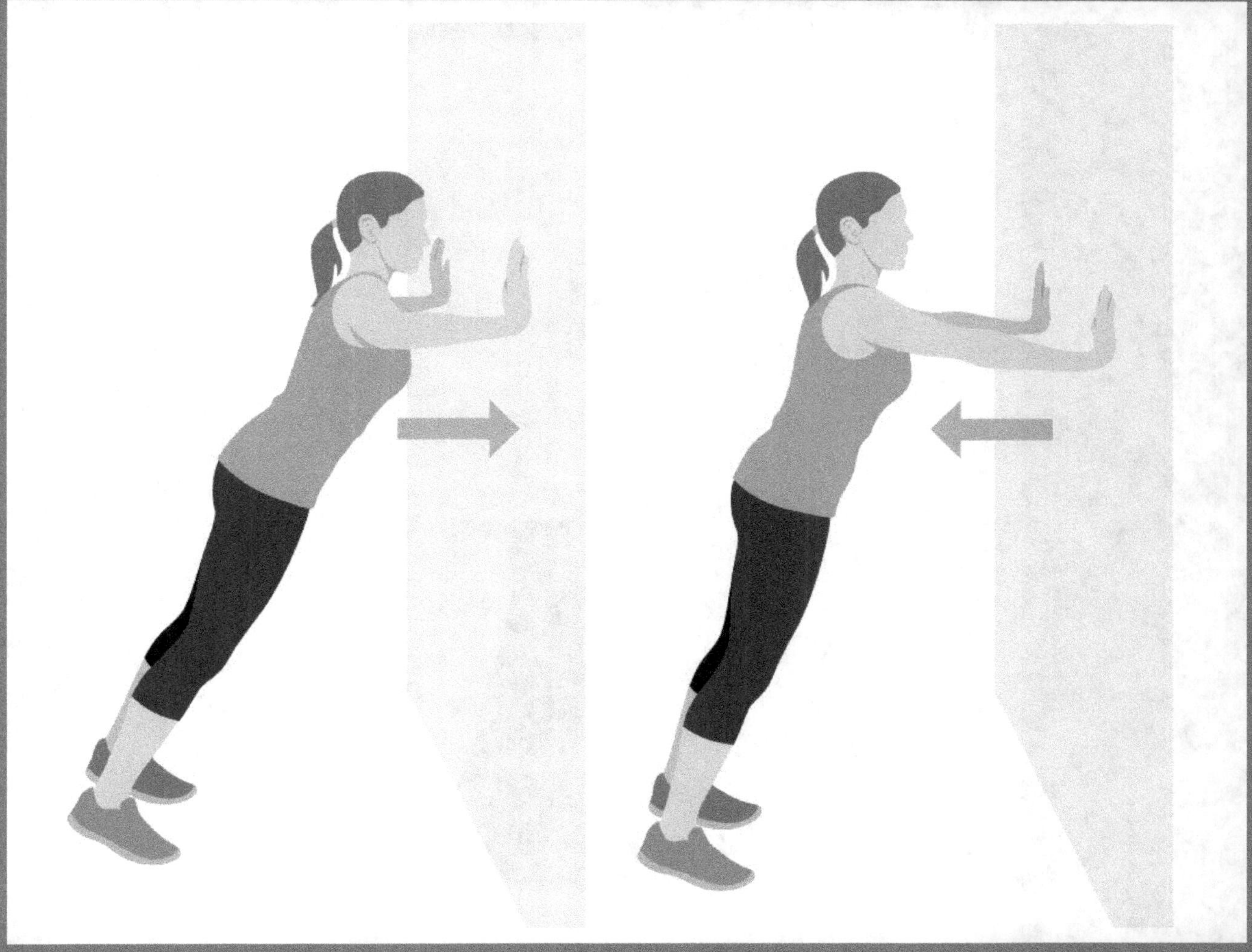

1. STAND FACING A WALL, ABOUT ARM'S LENGTH AWAY, WITH YOUR FEET HIP-WIDTH APART.
2. PLACE YOUR HANDS ON THE WALL SLIGHTLY WIDER THAN SHOULDER-WIDTH APART, AT SHOULDER HEIGHT OR SLIGHTLY LOWER.
3. DRAW YOUR NAVEL TOWARDS YOUR SPINE TO ENGAGE YOUR CORE MUSCLES.
4. EXHALE AS YOU BEND YOUR ELBOWS AND LOWER YOUR CHEST TOWARDS THE WALL, KEEPING YOUR BODY IN A STRAIGHT LINE FROM HEAD TO HEELS.
5. INHALE AS YOU PUSH THROUGH YOUR PALMS TO STRAIGHTEN YOUR ARMS, RETURNING TO THE STARTING POSITION.

BENEFITS: HELPS ENGAGE THE CHEST, SHOULDERS, AND TRICEPS WHILE PROVIDING SUPPORT FOR THE LOWER BACK AND CORE.

"YOU ARE DOING BETTER THAN YOU THINK."

28 DAY CHALLENGE:

5. TOE TAP CRUNCH

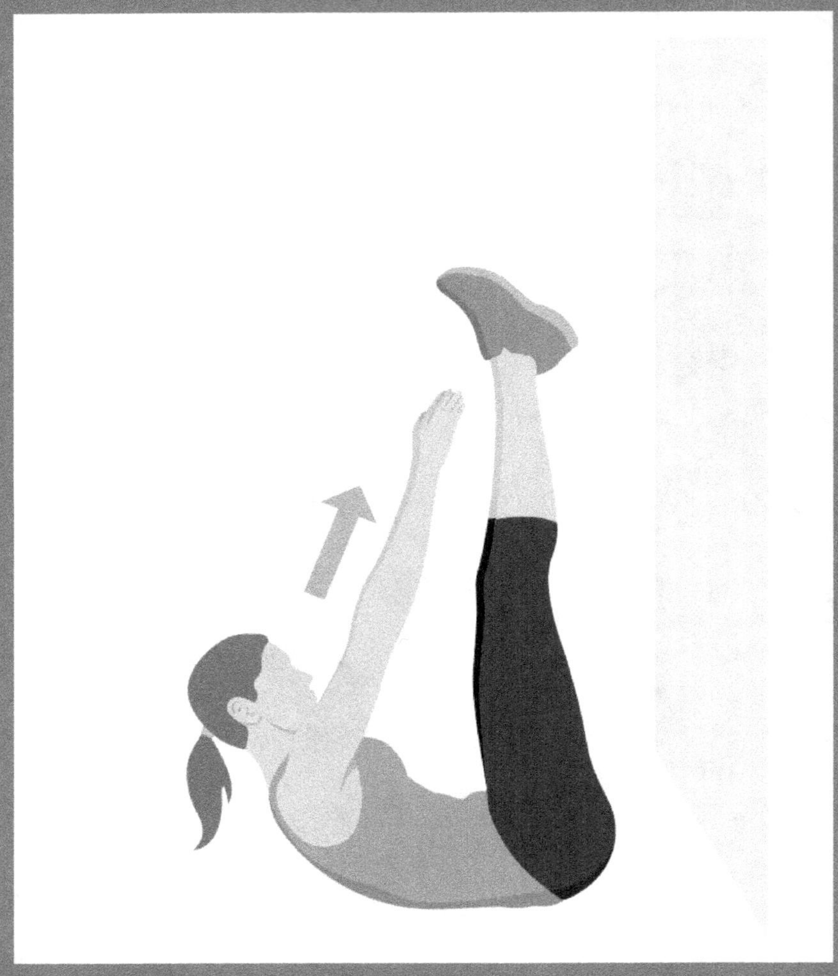

1. LIE ON YOUR BACK WITH YOUR LEGS EXTENDED VERTICALLY AGAINST A WALL AND YOUR ARMS BY YOUR SIDES.
2. DRAW YOUR NAVEL TOWARDS YOUR SPINE TO ENGAGE YOUR ABDOMINAL MUSCLES.
3. EXHALE AS YOU LIFT YOUR HEAD, NECK, AND SHOULDERS OFF THE MAT, AIMING TO TOUCH YOUR TOES WITH YOUR HANDS.
4. WHILE MAINTAINING THE CRUNCH POSITION, TAP YOUR TOES LIGHTLY AGAINST THE WALL, ALTERNATING BETWEEN LEGS.
5. HOLD THE CRUNCH POSITION BRIEFLY, FEELING THE CONTRACTION IN YOUR ABDOMINAL MUSCLES.
6. INHALE AS YOU LOWER YOUR UPPER BODY BACK TOWARDS THE MAT, KEEPING CONTROL OF THE MOVEMENT.

BENEFITS: HELPS TARGET THE ABDOMINAL MUSCLES EFFECTIVELY WHILE ALSO ENGAGING THE LOWER BODY MUSCLES.

"YOUR MIND, SOUL AND BODY ARE FULLY CONNECTED."

6. FROG CRUNCHES

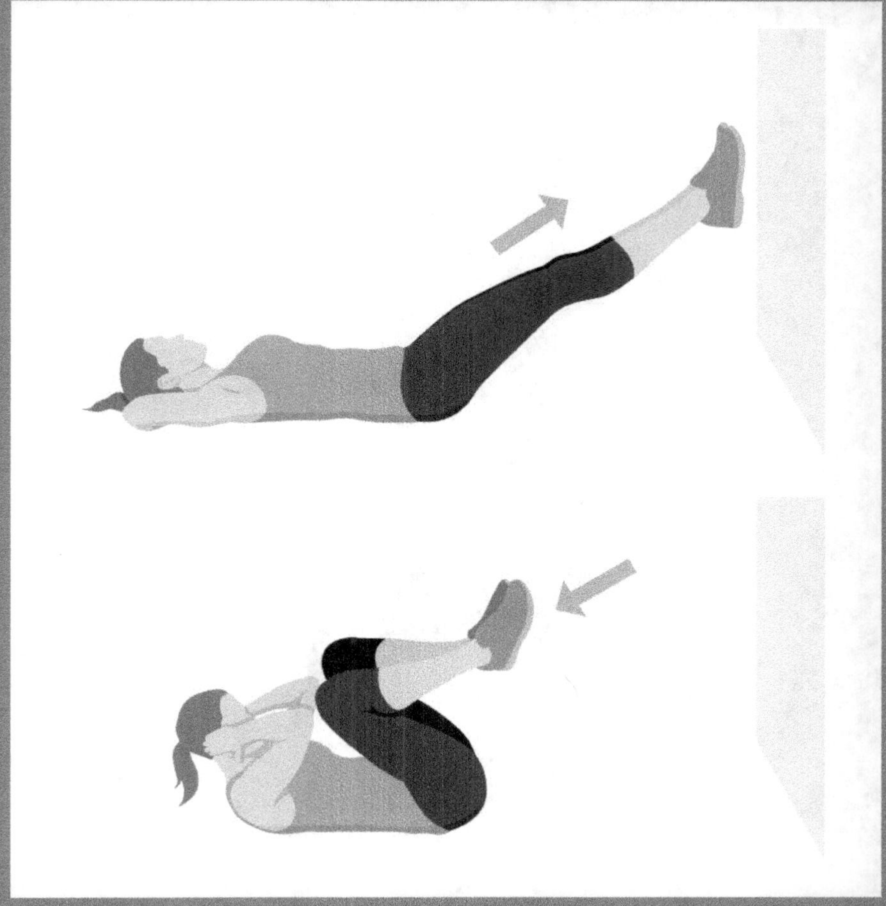

1. LIE ON YOUR BACK WITH YOUR FEET FLAT AGAINST A WALL, KNEES BENT, AND LEGS FORMING A DIAMOND SHAPE WITH SOLES OF THE FEET TOUCHING.
2. DRAW YOUR NAVEL(BELLY BUTTON) TOWARDS YOUR SPINE TO ENGAGE YOUR ABDOMINAL MUSCLES.
3. EXHALE AS YOU LIFT YOUR HEAD, NECK, AND SHOULDERS OFF THE MAT, AIMING TO BRING YOUR RIBCAGE TOWARDS YOUR HIPS.
4. HOLD THE CRUNCH POSITION BRIEFLY, FEELING THE CONTRACTION IN YOUR ABDOMINAL MUSCLES.
5. INHALE AS YOU SLOWLY LOWER YOUR UPPER BODY BACK TOWARDS THE MAT, KEEPING CONTROL OF THE MOVEMENT.

BENEFITS: HELPS TARGET THE ABDOMINAL MUSCLES EFFECTIVELY AND GREAT CORE STRENGTH AND STABILITY.

"YOU ARE FULL OF TREASURES."

7. 28 DAY CHALLENGE:
WALL SQUAT WITH LEG LIFT

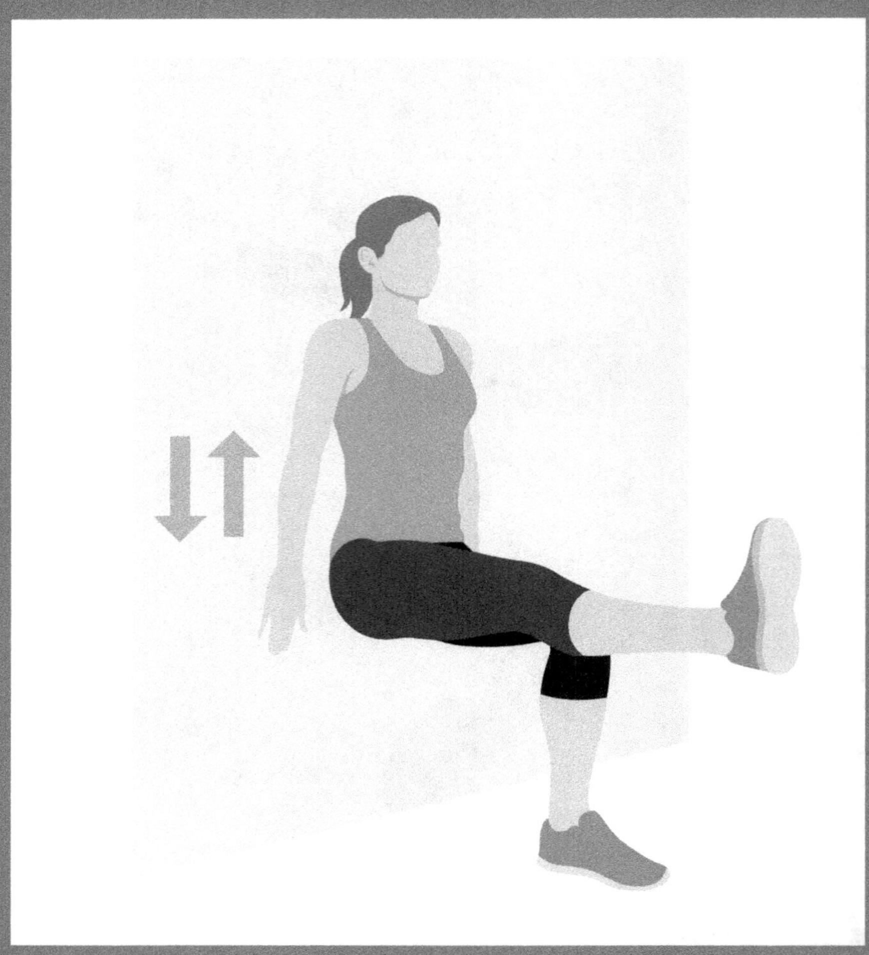

1. STAND WITH YOUR BACK AGAINST A WALL, FEET HIP-WIDTH APART, AND KNEES SLIGHTLY BENT.
2. DRAW YOUR BELLY BUTTON TOWARDS YOUR SPINE TO ENGAGE YOUR ABDOMINAL MUSCLES.
3. LOWER INTO A SQUAT POSITION BY SLIDING DOWN THE WALL, KEEPING YOUR BACK AGAINST IT AND KNEES ALIGNED WITH ANKLES.
4. AS YOU HOLD THE SQUAT, EXHALE AND LIFT ONE LEG STRAIGHT OUT IN FRONT OF YOU, KEEPING IT PARALLEL TO THE GROUND.
5. HOLD THE LEG LIFT BRIEFLY, FEELING THE ENGAGEMENT IN YOUR CORE AND LEG MUSCLES. THEN, LOWER THE LEG BACK DOWN.
6. REPEAT THE LEG LIFTS ON THE OPPOSITE SIDE, ENSURING TO MAINTAIN PROPER FORM AND BALANCE.

BENEFITS: HELPS STRENGTHEN YOUR LOWER BODY, IMPROVES CORE STABILITY, AND ENHANCES BALANCE AND COORDINATION.

"YOU ARE RIGHT AROUND THE CORNER. DON'T GIVE UP."

28 DAY CHALLENGE:

8. SIDE PLANK HIP OPENER – RIGHT/LEFT

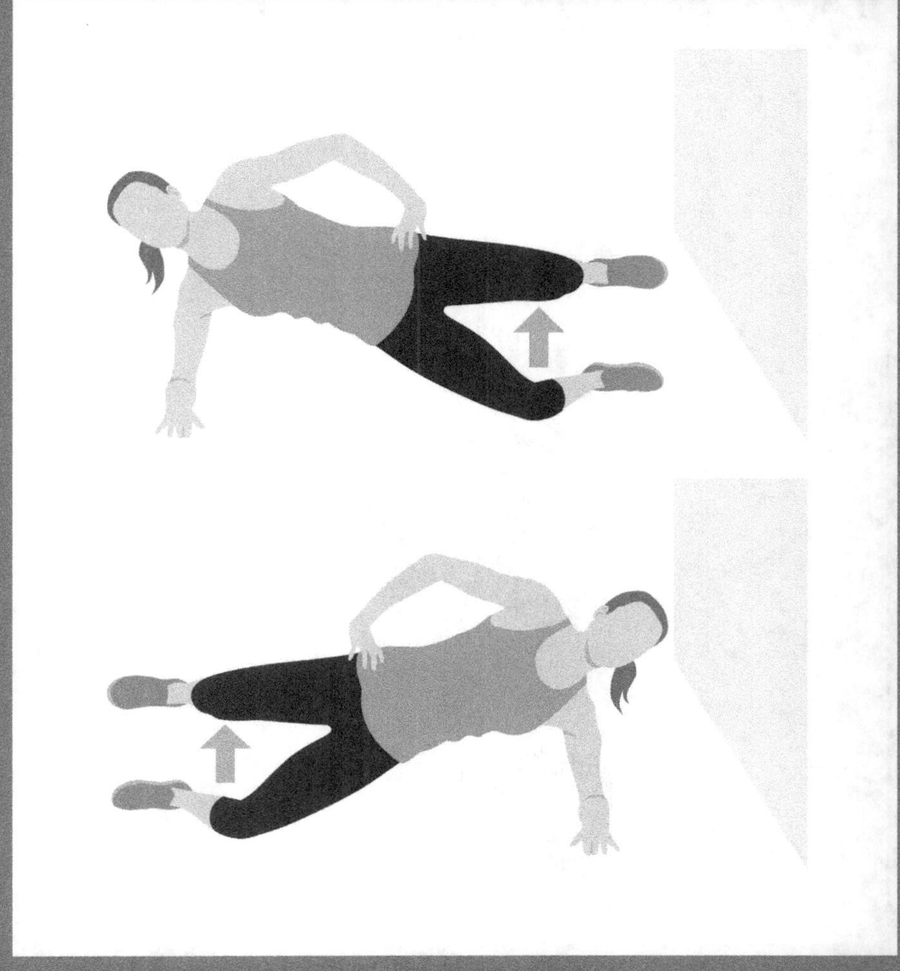

1. BEGIN IN A SIDE PLANK POSITION WITH YOUR RIGHT SIDE FACING THE WALL, FOREARM ON THE MAT, AND FEET STACKED.
2. DRAW YOUR NAVEL TOWARDS YOUR SPINE TO ENGAGE YOUR CORE MUSCLES.
3. LIFT YOUR HIPS OFF THE MAT, CREATING A STRAIGHT LINE FROM HEAD TO HEELS.
4. EXHALE AS YOU ROTATE YOUR TORSO TOWARDS THE WALL, OPENING YOUR CHEST AND HIPS UPWARD. EXTEND YOUR TOP ARM TOWARDS THE CEILING FOR BALANCE.
5. HOLD THE POSITION BRIEFLY, FEELING THE STRETCH THROUGH YOUR CHEST, SHOULDERS, AND HIPS.
6. INHALE AS YOU GENTLY ROTATE YOUR TORSO BACK TO THE STARTING SIDE PLANK POSITION.
7. SWITCH TO THE LEFT SIDE, PERFORMING THE SIDE PLANK WITH HIP OPENER ON THE OPPOSITE SIDE.

BENEFITS: HELPS STRENGTHENS THE CORE, INCREASES HIP MOBILITY, ENHANCES SHOULDER STABILITY AND IMPROVES POSTURE, BALANCE.

"YOU ARE STRONGER THAT YOU THINK."

28 DAY CHALLENGE:

9. HIP OPENER TO LEG EXTEND – RIGHT/LEFT

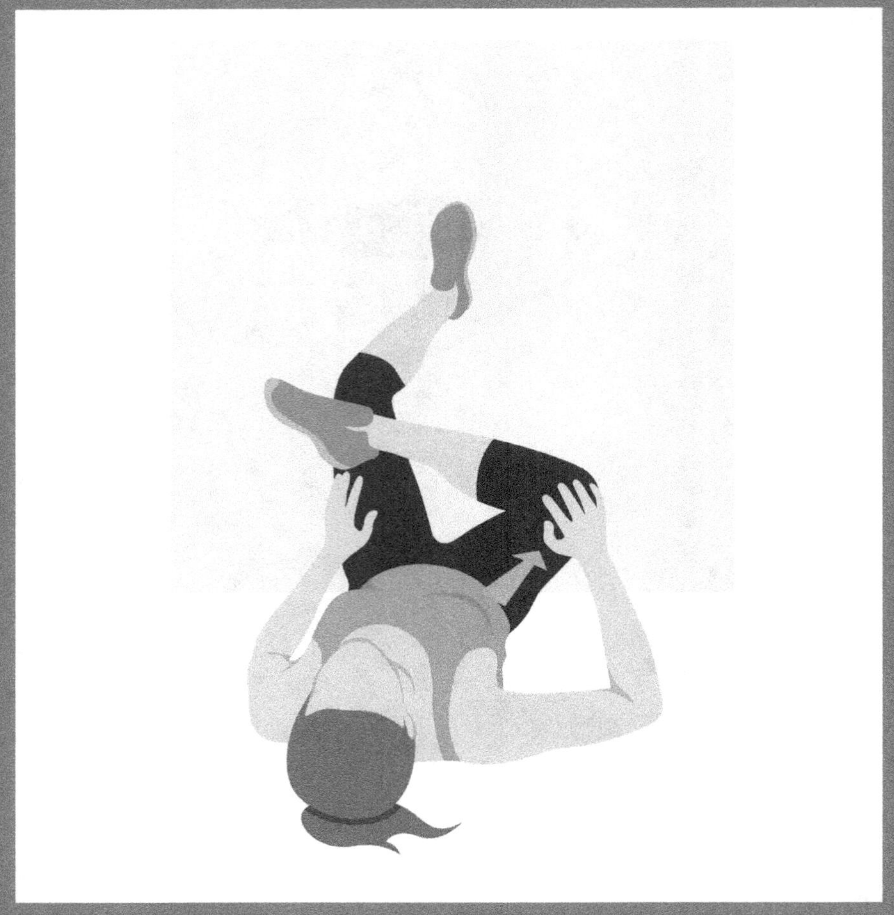

1. BEGIN IN A SIDE PLANK POSITION WITH YOUR RIGHT SIDE FACING THE WALL, FOREARM ON THE MAT, AND FEET STACKED.
2. DRAW YOUR NAVEL TOWARDS YOUR SPINE TO ENGAGE YOUR CORE MUSCLES.
3. EXHALE AS YOU ROTATE YOUR TORSO TOWARDS THE WALL, OPENING YOUR CHEST AND HIPS UPWARD.
4. INHALE AS YOU EXTEND YOUR TOP LEG STRAIGHT OUT IN FRONT OF YOU, KEEPING IT IN LINE WITH YOUR BODY.
5. HOLD THE POSITION BRIEFLY, FEELING THE STRETCH THROUGH YOUR CHEST, SHOULDERS, AND HIP FLEXORS, WHILE ENGAGING YOUR CORE TO STABILIZE.
6. EXHALE AS YOU GENTLY RETURN TO THE SIDE PLANK POSITION WITH YOUR LEG LIFTED.

BENEFITS: HELPS STRENGTHENS THE CORE, IMPROVES HIP FLEXIBILITY, AND ENHANCES SHOULDER STABILITY.

"VISUALIZE YOUR END GOAL AND KEEP PRESSING INTO IT"

28 DAY CHALLENGE:

10.   RAINBOWS

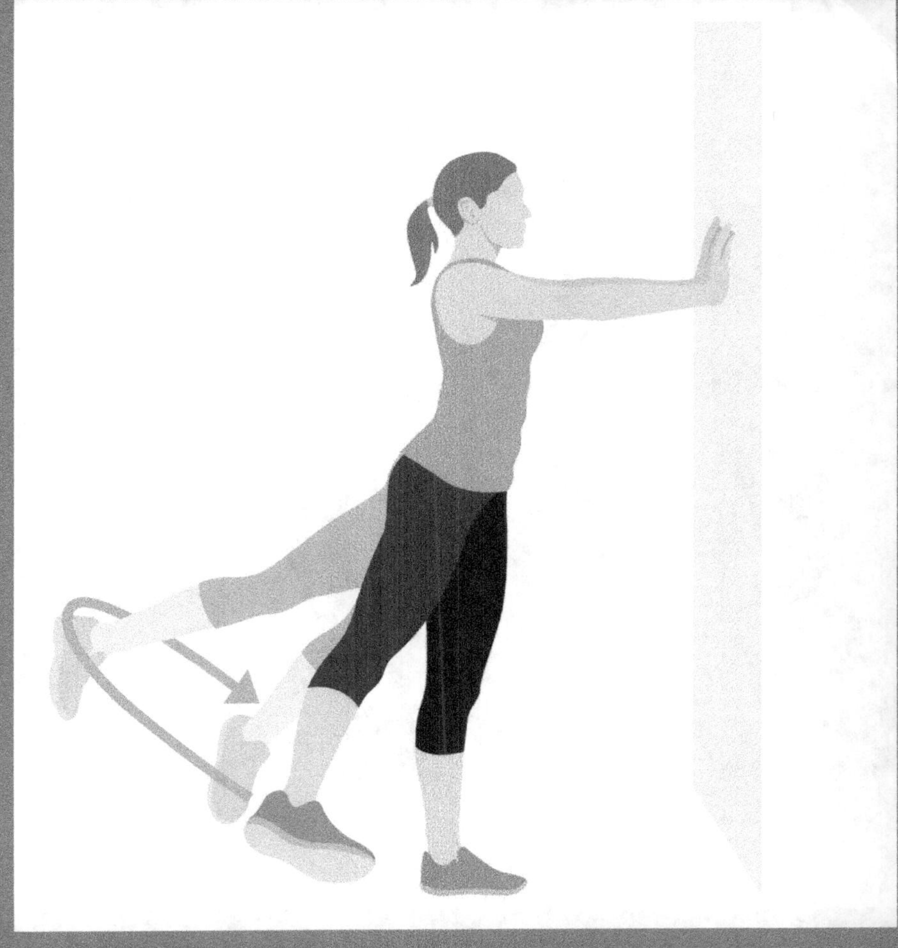

1. STAND FACING A WALL WITH YOUR FEET HIP-WIDTH APART AND YOUR ARMS EXTENDED OVERHEAD, PALMS PRESSING AGAINST THE WALL.
2. DRAW YOUR BELLY BUTTON TOWARDS YOUR SPINE TO ENGAGE YOUR ABDOMINAL MUSCLES.
3. EXHALE AS YOU TRACE A RAINBOW SHAPE WITH YOUR HANDS, LOWERING THEM TO ONE SIDE IN A SWEEPING MOTION TOWARDS THE FLOOR, THEN BACK UP AND OVER TO THE OPPOSITE SIDE.
4. AS YOU MOVE YOUR ARMS, SHIFT YOUR WEIGHT SLIGHTLY ONTO THE OPPOSITE LEG TO MAINTAIN BALANCE AND STABILITY.
5. FOCUS ON FEELING THE STRETCH THROUGH YOUR SIDE BODY AS YOU REACH TOWARDS THE FLOOR.
6. INHALE AS YOU BRING YOUR ARMS BACK TO THE CENTER, RETURNING TO THE STARTING POSITION WITH CONTROL.

BENEFITS: HELPS ENGAGE THE CORE, STRETCHES THE SIDES, AND INCREASES SHOULDER MOBILITY, OFFERING A DYNAMIC WORKOUT FOR OVERALL STRENGTH AND FLEXIBILITY.

"BE NICE TO YOURSELF."

28 DAY CHALLENGE:

11. WALL PLANK WITH SHOULDER TAPS

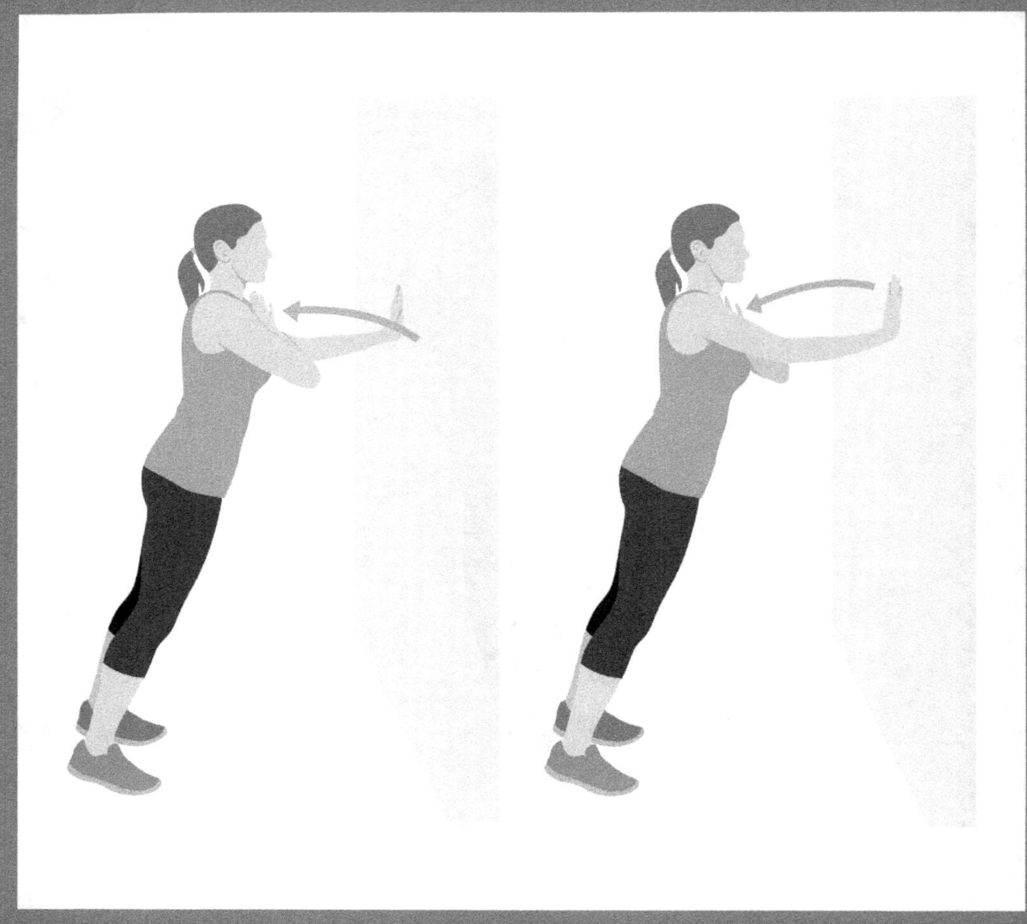

1. BEGIN IN A PLANK POSITION FACING THE WALL, WITH YOUR HANDS SHOULDER-WIDTH APART AND YOUR FEET HIP-WIDTH APART.
2. DRAW YOUR BELLY BUTTON TOWARDS YOUR SPINE TO ENGAGE YOUR ABDOMINAL MUSCLES AND MAINTAIN A STRAIGHT LINE FROM HEAD TO HEELS.
3. LIFT ONE HAND OFF THE FLOOR AND TAP THE OPPOSITE SHOULDER, KEEPING YOUR HIPS AND TORSO STABLE.
4. RETURN THE HAND TO THE FLOOR AND TAP THE OTHER SHOULDER WITH THE OPPOSITE HAND, MAINTAINING STABILITY THROUGHOUT.

BENEFITS: HELPS STRENGTHEN THE CORE, SHOULDERS, AND STABILIZING MUSCLES, IMPROVING BALANCE AND BODY AWARENESS.

"YOUR DREAMS ARE CLOSER THAN YOU THINK."

12.

WALL BRIDGE WITH MARCHING

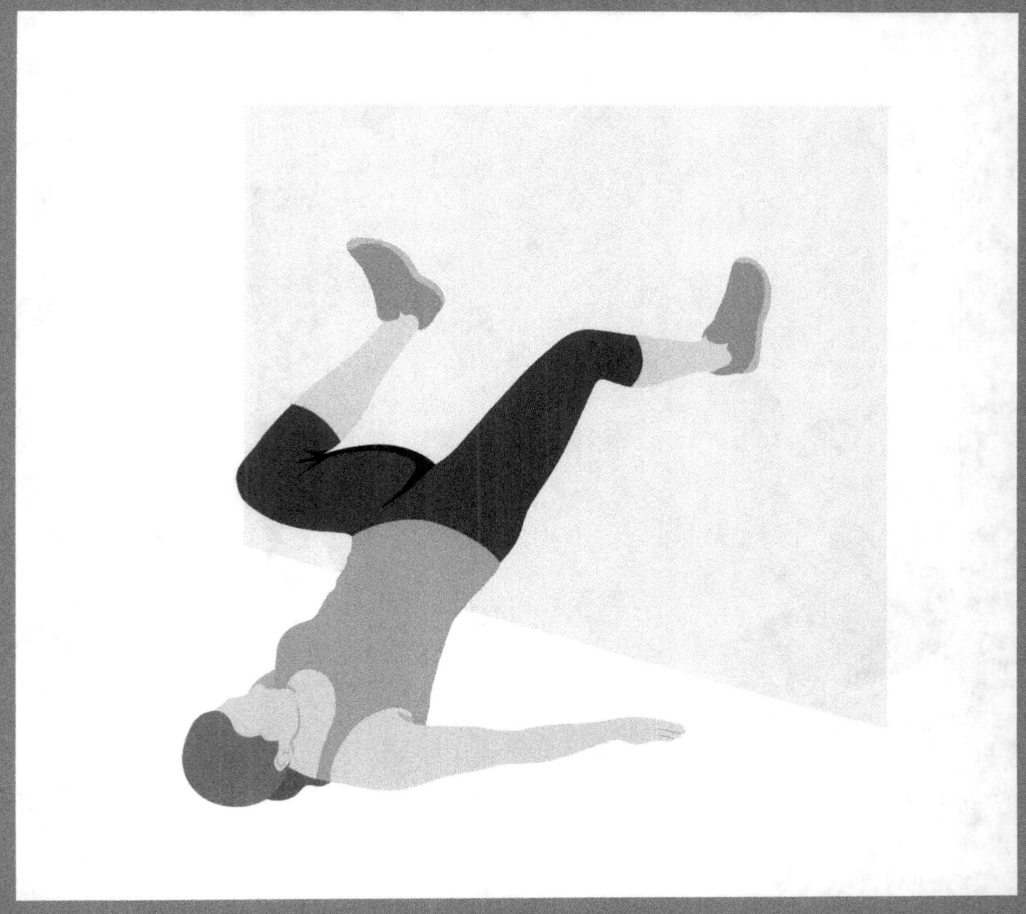

1. LIE ON YOUR BACK WITH YOUR FEET FLAT AGAINST A WALL, KNEES BENT, AND ARMS BY YOUR SIDES.
2. DRAW YOUR NAVEL TOWARDS YOUR SPINE TO ENGAGE YOUR ABDOMINAL MUSCLES.
3. EXHALE AS YOU LIFT YOUR HIPS OFF THE MAT, FORMING A BRIDGE POSITION, WITH YOUR BODY IN A STRAIGHT LINE FROM SHOULDERS TO KNEES.
4. WHILE MAINTAINING THE BRIDGE POSITION, LIFT ONE KNEE TOWARDS YOUR CHEST, THEN LOWER IT BACK DOWN. ALTERNATE LEGS, MARCHING IN PLACE.
5. HOLD THE BRIDGE POSITION AND FEEL THE ENGAGEMENT IN YOUR GLUTES AND CORE MUSCLES AS YOU MARCH.
6. INHALE AS YOU LOWER YOUR HIPS BACK DOWN TO THE MAT, RETURNING TO THE STARTING POSITION WITH CONTROL.

BENEFITS: HELPS ENHANCE LOWER BODY STRENGTH, CORE STABILITY, AND COORDINATION, PROMOTING OVERALL FUNCTIONAL FITNESS.

"YOU ARE HEALTHY. "

28 DAY CHALLENGE:

13. JUMPING WALL SQUATS

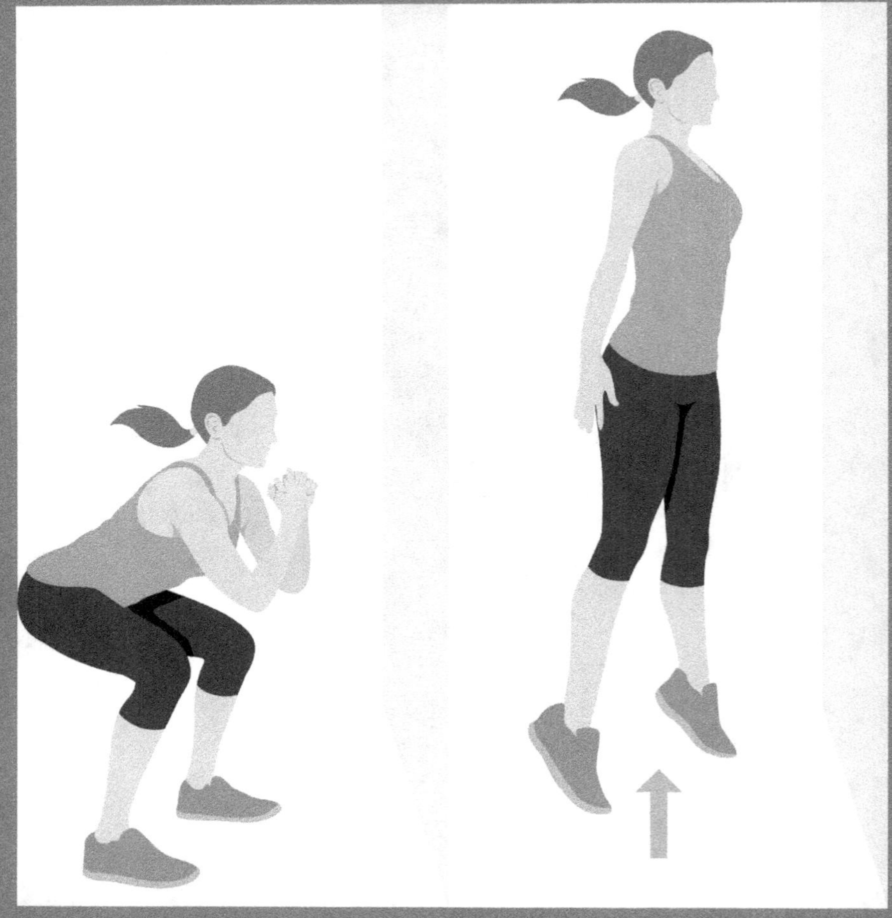

1. STAND FACING A WALL WITH YOUR FEET HIP-WIDTH APART AND YOUR ARMS BY YOUR SIDES.
2. DRAW YOUR NAVEL TOWARDS YOUR SPINE TO ENGAGE YOUR ABDOMINAL MUSCLES.
3. BEND YOUR KNEES AND LOWER INTO A SQUAT POSITION, KEEPING YOUR BACK STRAIGHT AND CHEST LIFTED.
4. PUSH THROUGH YOUR FEET AND JUMP EXPLOSIVELY, AIMING TO REACH YOUR HANDS UP TOWARDS THE WALL.
5. LAND BACK INTO THE SQUAT POSITION WITH CONTROL, ENSURING TO ABSORB THE IMPACT WITH YOUR LEGS.

BENEFITS: HELPS ELEVATE HEART RATE AND STRENGTHEN LOWER BODY MUSCLES, PROVIDING A DYNAMIC WORKOUT THAT ENHANCES POWER AND AGILITY.

14. EXPLOSIVE WALL PUSH-UPS

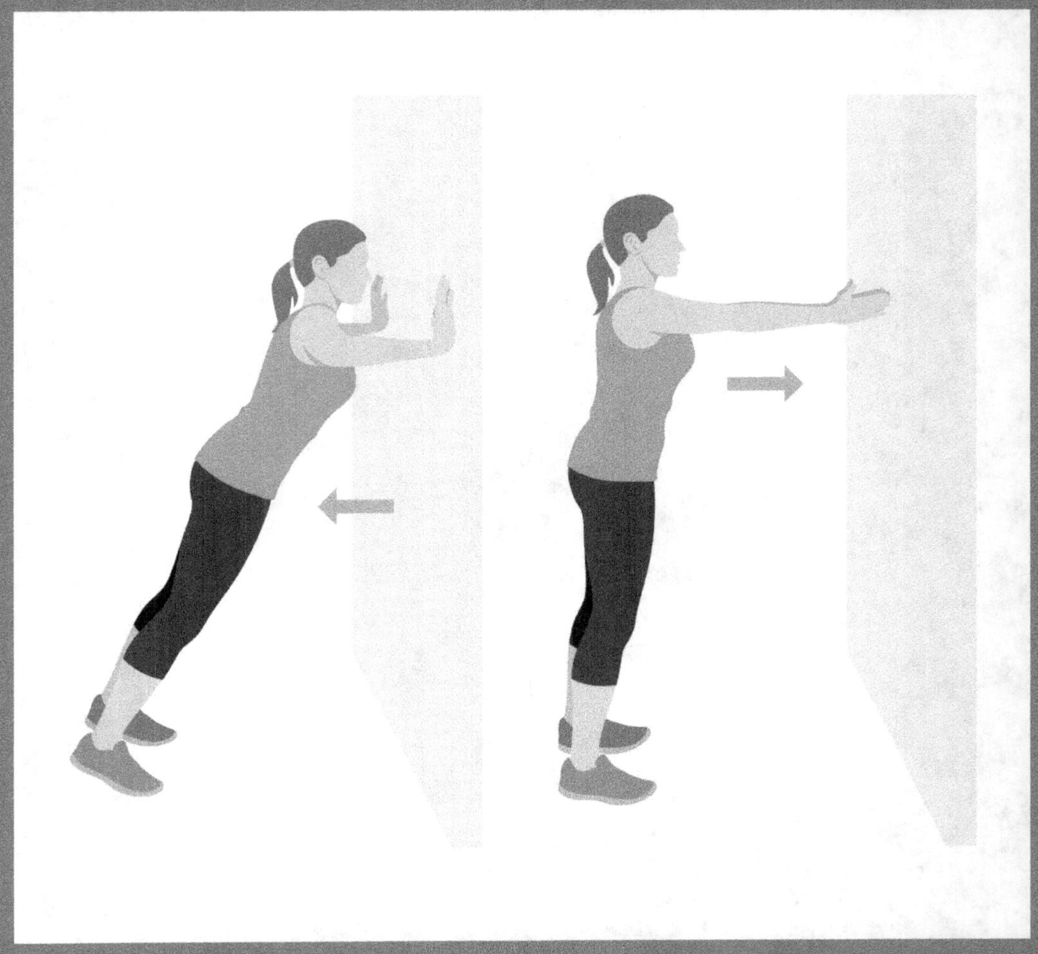

1. STAND FACING A WALL WITH YOUR ARMS EXTENDED, PALMS FLAT AGAINST THE WALL AT SHOULDER HEIGHT OR SLIGHTLY LOWER.
2. DRAW YOUR NAVEL TOWARDS YOUR SPINE TO ENGAGE YOUR ABDOMINAL MUSCLES.
3. LOWER YOUR CHEST TOWARDS THE WALL BY BENDING YOUR ELBOWS, THEN EXPLOSIVELY PUSH AWAY FROM THE WALL, PROPELLING YOUR HANDS OFF THE WALL.
4. LAND SOFTLY AND ABSORB THE IMPACT BY BENDING YOUR ELBOWS SLIGHTLY AS YOU BRING YOUR HANDS BACK TO THE WALL.

BENEFITS: HELPS ENGAGE UPPER BODY MUSCLES AND ENHANCE POWER AND COORDINATION, OFFERING AN EFFECTIVE WAY TO STRENGTHEN AND TONE THE ARMS, SHOULDERS, AND CHEST.

"YOUR BODY NEEDS YOU."

28 DAY CHALLENGE:
15. WALL PLANK WITH KNEE DRIVES

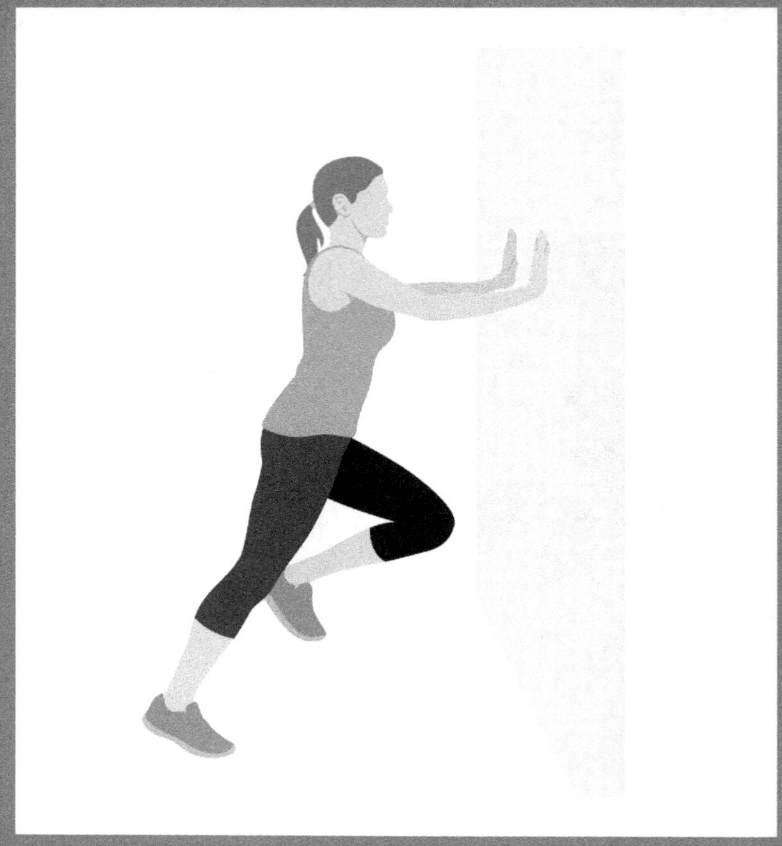

1. BEGIN IN A PLANK POSITION FACING THE WALL, WITH YOUR HANDS SHOULDER-WIDTH APART AND YOUR FEET HIP-WIDTH APART.
2. DRAW YOUR NAVEL TOWARDS YOUR SPINE TO ENGAGE YOUR ABDOMINAL MUSCLES AND MAINTAIN A STRAIGHT LINE FROM HEAD TO HEELS.
3. EXHALE AS YOU LIFT ONE KNEE TOWARDS YOUR CHEST, AIMING TO BRING IT AS CLOSE TO YOUR HANDS AS POSSIBLE WHILE MAINTAINING STABILITY.
4. INHALE AS YOU EXTEND THE LIFTED LEG BACK TO THE STARTING PLANK POSITION, KEEPING YOUR HIPS STABLE AND CORE ENGAGED.
5. REPEAT THE KNEE DRIVE MOVEMENT ON THE OPPOSITE SIDE, FOCUSING ON CONTROLLED MOVEMENTS AND KEEPING YOUR CORE TIGHT.

BENEFITS: HELPS ENGAGE THE CORE AND IMPROVES STABILITY WHILE ENHANCING LOWER BODY STRENGTH AND COORDINATION, PROVIDING A DYNAMIC AND EFFECTIVE FULL-BODY WORKOUT.

"HEALTH BELONGS TO YOU."

28 DAY CHALLENGE:

16. WALL BRIDGE WITH ALTERNATING LEG EXTENSIONS

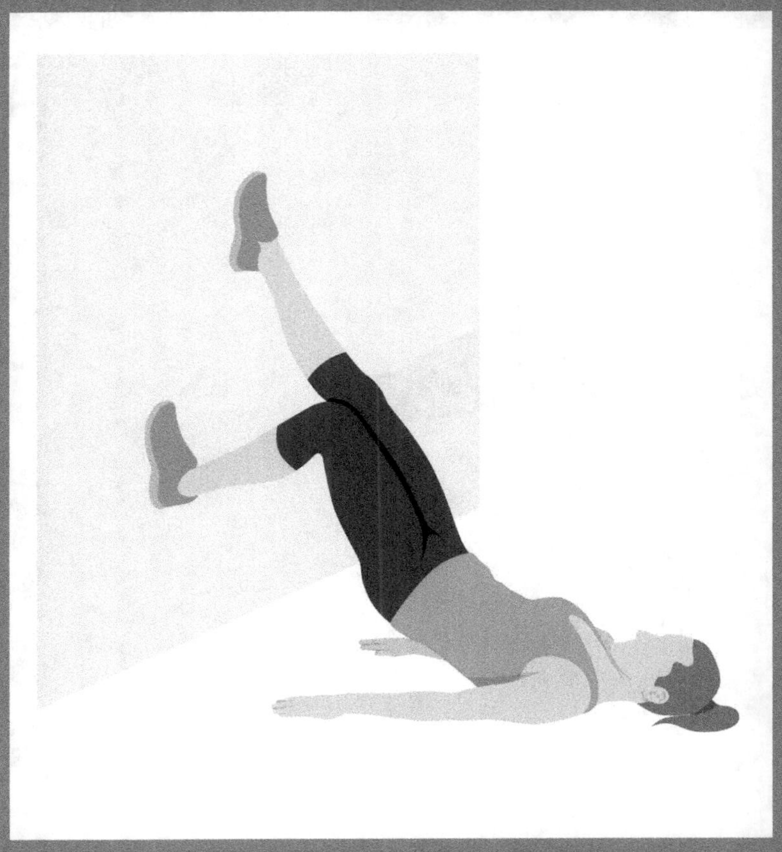

1. LIE ON YOUR BACK WITH YOUR FEET FLAT AGAINST A WALL, KNEES BENT, AND ARMS BY YOUR SIDES.
2. DRAW YOUR NAVEL TOWARDS YOUR SPINE TO ENGAGE YOUR ABDOMINAL MUSCLES.
3. EXHALE AS YOU LIFT YOUR HIPS OFF THE MAT, FORMING A BRIDGE POSITION, WITH YOUR BODY IN A STRAIGHT LINE FROM SHOULDERS TO KNEES.
4. WHILE MAINTAINING THE BRIDGE POSITION, EXTEND ONE LEG STRAIGHT OUT IN FRONT OF YOU, KEEPING IT IN LINE WITH YOUR BODY. ALTERNATE LEGS WITH CONTROL.
5. HOLD THE BRIDGE POSITION AND FEEL THE ENGAGEMENT IN YOUR GLUTES AND CORE MUSCLES AS YOU EXTEND YOUR LEGS.
6. INHALE AS YOU LOWER YOUR HIPS BACK DOWN TO THE MAT, RETURNING TO THE STARTING POSITION WITH CONTROL.

BENEFITS: HELP ENHANCE LOWER BODY STRENGTH, CORE STABILITY, AND COORDINATION, PROVIDING A COMPREHENSIVE WORKOUT FOR OVERALL FITNESS AND MUSCLE TONING.

"WELL-BEING IS YOUR PORTION."

28 DAY CHALLENGE:

17. WALL PIKE PRESS

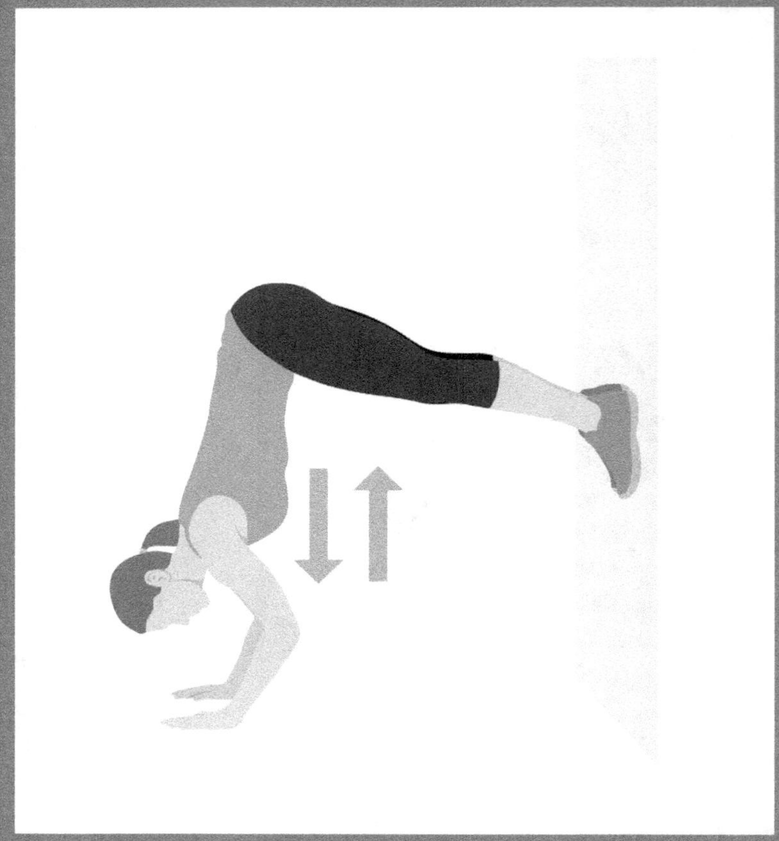

1. BEGIN IN A PLANK POSITION FACING THE WALL, WITH YOUR HANDS SHOULDER-WIDTH APART AND YOUR FEET HIP-WIDTH APART.
2. DRAW YOUR NAVEL TOWARDS YOUR SPINE TO ENGAGE YOUR ABDOMINAL MUSCLES AND MAINTAIN A STRAIGHT LINE FROM HEAD TO HEELS.
3. EXHALE AS YOU LIFT YOUR HIPS TOWARDS THE CEILING, FORMING AN INVERTED V SHAPE WITH YOUR BODY.
4. PRESS YOUR HANDS FIRMLY INTO THE WALL, FOCUSING ON ENGAGING YOUR SHOULDERS AND UPPER BACK MUSCLES.
5. HOLD THE PIKE POSITION BRIEFLY, FEELING THE STRETCH THROUGH YOUR HAMSTRINGS AND SHOULDERS.
6. INHALE AS YOU LOWER YOUR HIPS BACK DOWN TO THE STARTING PLANK POSITION WITH CONTROL.

BENEFITS: HELP STRENGTHEN THE SHOULDERS, UPPER BACK, AND CORE WHILE IMPROVING SHOULDER MOBILITY AND FLEXIBILITY, PROVIDING A COMPREHENSIVE UPPER BODY WORKOUT.

28 DAY CHALLENGE:

18. WALL SQUAT TO BUTTERFLY CRUNCH

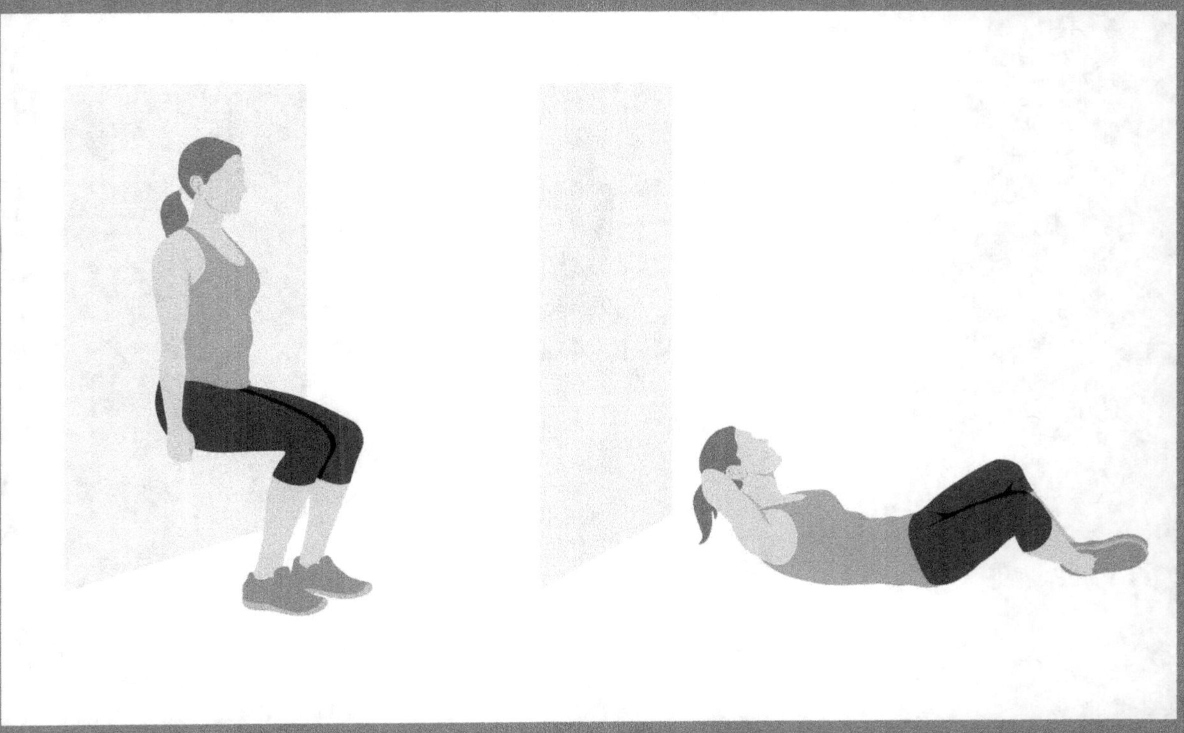

1. STAND WITH YOUR BACK AGAINST A WALL AND YOUR FEET HIP-WIDTH APART.
2. LOWER INTO A SQUAT POSITION, SLIDING DOWN THE WALL UNTIL YOUR THIGHS ARE PARALLEL TO THE GROUND.
3. DRAW YOUR NAVEL TOWARDS YOUR SPINE TO ENGAGE YOUR ABDOMINAL MUSCLES.
4. AS YOU HOLD THE SQUAT POSITION, BRING YOUR KNEES TOGETHER AND OPEN YOUR THIGHS OUTWARD, RESEMBLING A BUTTERFLY POSITION. SIMULTANEOUSLY, PERFORM A CRUNCH BY BRINGING YOUR ELBOWS TOWARDS YOUR KNEES, ENGAGING YOUR CORE.
5. SLOWLY RETURN TO THE STANDING POSITION, STRAIGHTENING YOUR LEGS AND BRINGING YOUR ARMS BACK DOWN BY YOUR SIDES.

BENEFITS: HELPS COMBINE LOWER BODY STRENGTH TRAINING WITH CORE ENGAGEMENT, PROMOTING MUSCLE TONING, IMPROVED POSTURE, AND ENHANCED FLEXIBILITY.

28 DAY CHALLENGE:

19. SINGLE LEG GLUTE BRIDGE TO TOE TAP CRUNCH

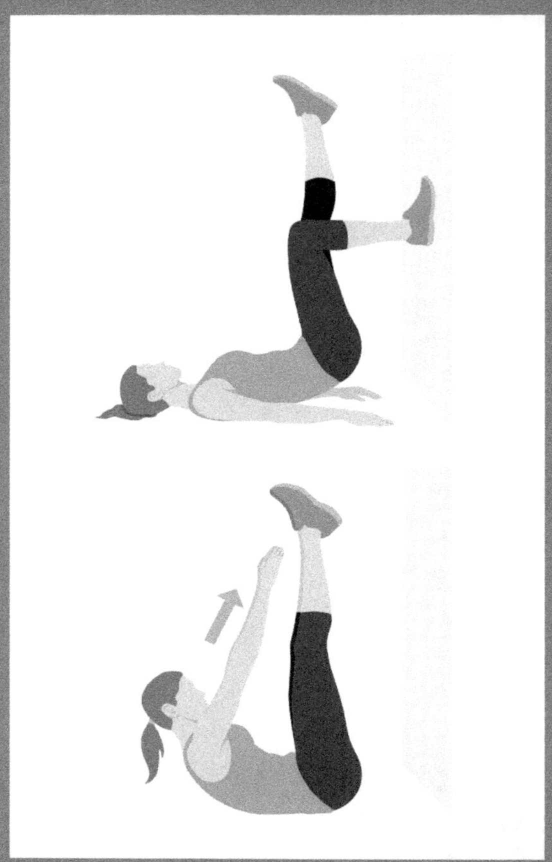

1. LIE ON YOUR BACK WITH YOUR FEET FLAT AGAINST A WALL, KNEES BENT, AND ARMS BY YOUR SIDES.
2. LIFT YOUR HIPS OFF THE MAT, FORMING A BRIDGE POSITION, WHILE EXTENDING ONE LEG STRAIGHT UP TOWARDS THE CEILING.
3. CRUNCH UPWARDS, REACHING YOUR OPPOSITE HAND TOWARDS THE LIFTED FOOT WHILE TAPPING IT LIGHTLY, ENGAGING YOUR CORE.
4. HOLD THE POSITION BRIEFLY, FEELING THE CONTRACTION IN YOUR ABDOMINAL MUSCLES.
5. LOWER YOUR UPPER BODY AND HIPS BACK DOWN TO THE MAT WITH CONTROL.

BENEFITS: HELPS COMBINES LOWER BODY STRENGTHENING WITH CORE ENGAGEMENT, ENHANCING STABILITY, BALANCE, AND OVERALL CORE STRENGTH FOR IMPROVED FUNCTIONAL FITNESS.

"LOVE ON YOUR BODY"

28 DAY CHALLENGE:

20. CRUNCHES TO FROG CRUNCHES SUPERSET

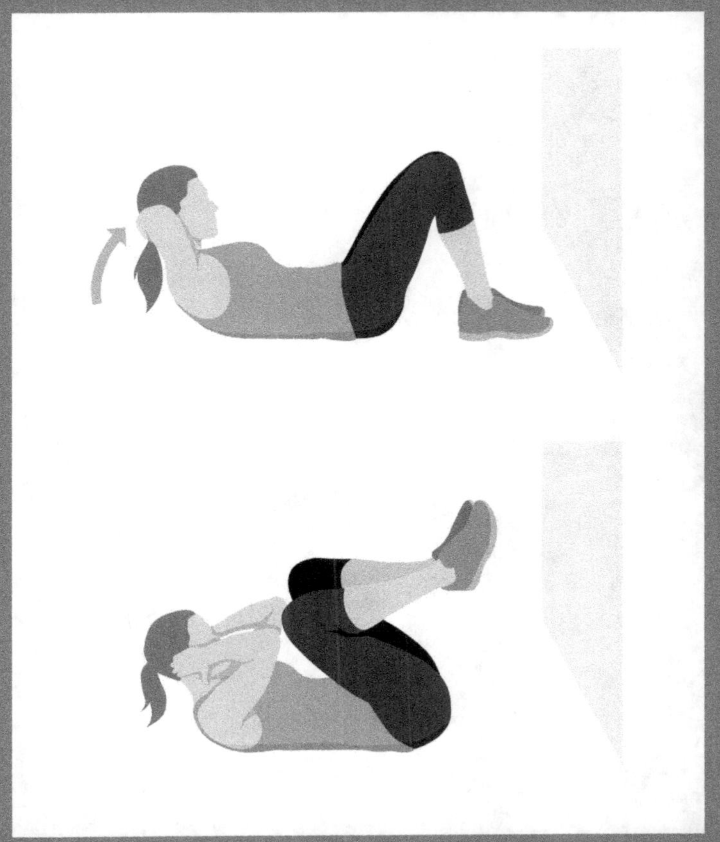

1. BEGIN LYING ON YOUR BACK WITH YOUR FEET FLAT AGAINST A WALL, KNEES BENT, AND ARMS BY YOUR SIDES.
2. EXHALE AS YOU LIFT YOUR HEAD, NECK, AND SHOULDERS OFF THE MAT, AIMING TO BRING YOUR RIBCAGE TOWARDS YOUR HIPS IN A TRADITIONAL CRUNCH MOVEMENT.
3. FROM THE CRUNCH POSITION, EXTEND YOUR ARMS AND LEGS OUTWARDS, THEN EXHALE AS YOU BRING YOUR KNEES TOWARDS YOUR CHEST AND YOUR ELBOWS TOWARDS YOUR KNEES, MIMICKING A FROG-LIKE MOTION.
4. INHALE AS YOU LOWER YOUR UPPER BODY AND LEGS BACK DOWN TO THE MAT WITH CONTROL.

BENEFITS: HELPS ENGAGE THE CORE MUSCLES THROUGH VARYING MOVEMENTS, FOSTERING ABDOMINAL STRENGTH, FLEXIBILITY, AND FUNCTIONAL STABILITY FOR OVERALL FITNESS ENHANCEMENT.

"CHOOSE ONE PART ON YOUR BODY AND SAY WHAT YOU LIKE ABOUT IT "

28 DAY CHALLENGE:

21. WALL PUSH-UPS TO SIDE PLANK HIP OPENER SUPERSET

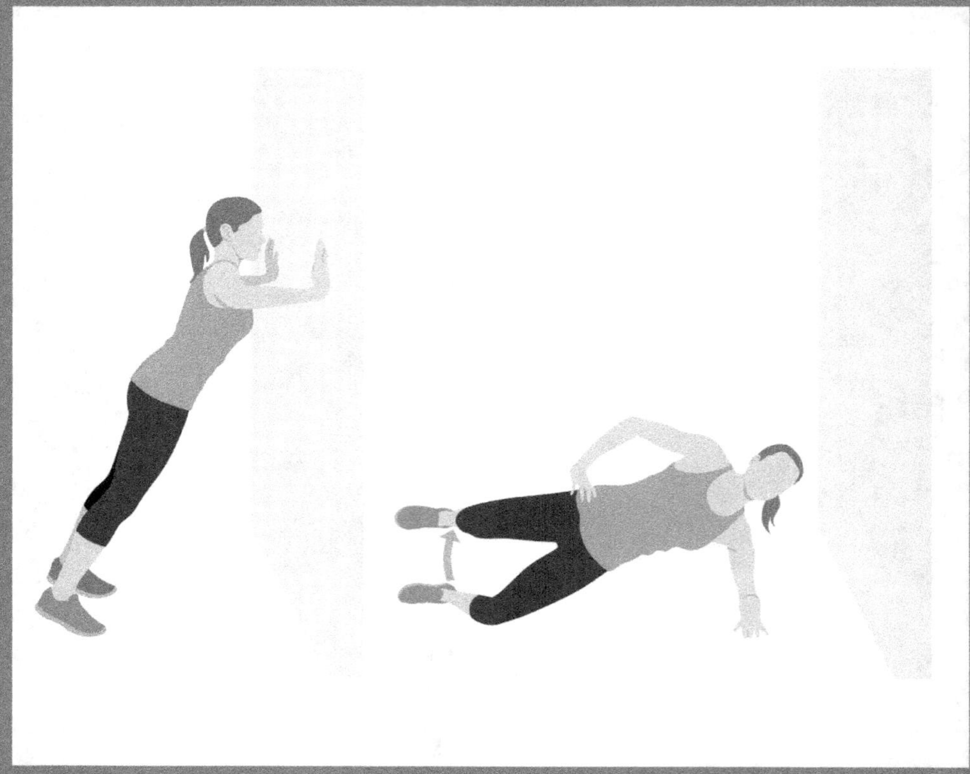

1. BEGIN IN A PUSH-UP POSITION FACING THE WALL, WITH YOUR HANDS SHOJLDER-WIDTH APART AND YOUR FEET HIP-WIDTH APART.
2. EXHALE AS YOU LOWER YOUR CHEST TOWARDS THE WALL BY BENDING YOUR ELBOWS, THEN PUSH AWAY FROM THE WALL TO RETURN TO THE STARTING POSITION.
3. FROM THE PUSH-UP POSITION, ROTATE YOUR BODY TO THE SIDE AND LIFT ONE ARM TOWARDS THE CEILING, COMING INTO A SIDE PLANK POSITION.
4. EXHALE AS YOU OPEN YOUR TOP HIP TOWARDS THE CEILING, STRETCHING THROUGH THE SIDE OF YOUR BODY.
5. INHALE AS YOU ROTATE BACK TO THE PUSH-UP POSITION, THEN REPEAT THE SEQUENCE ON THE OPPOSITE SIDE.

BENEFITS: HELPS INTEGRATE UPPER BODY STRENGTH AND CORE STABILITY EXERCISES, FOSTERING FUNCTIONAL STRENGTH, ENHANCED SHOULDER MOBILITY, AND OVERALL BODY COORDINATION.

22.

TOE TAP CRUNCH TO HIP OPENER TO LEG EXTEND – SUPERSET

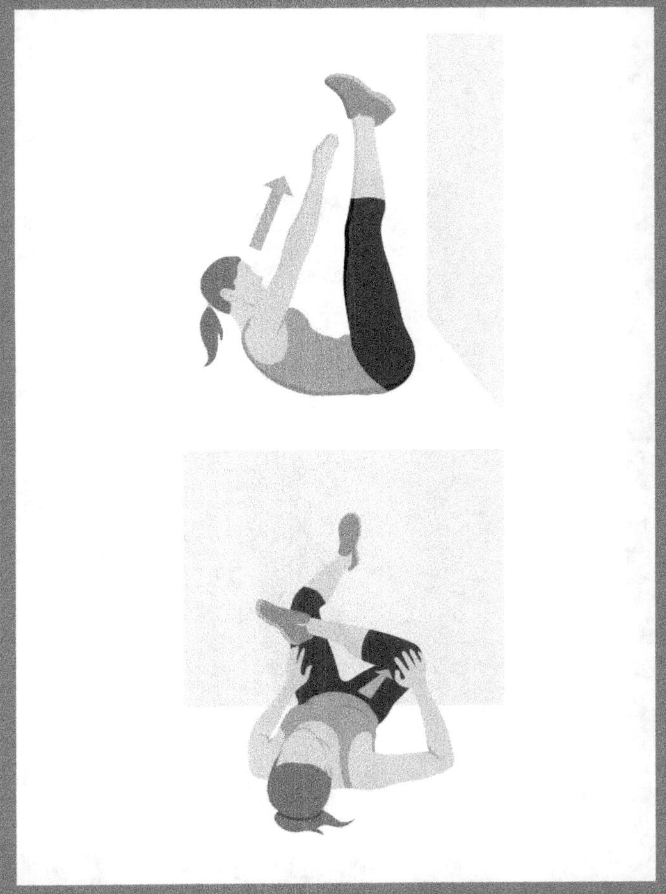

1. BEGIN LYING ON YOUR BACK WITH YOUR FEET FLAT AGAINST A WALL, KNEES BENT, AND ARMS BY YOUR SIDES.
2. EXHALE AS YOU LIFT YOUR HEAD, NECK, AND SHOULDERS OFF THE MAT, AIMING TO TOUCH YOUR TOES WITH YOUR HANDS WHILE TAPPING ONE FOOT LIGHTLY AGAINST THE WALL.
3. FROM THE CRUNCH POSITION, OPEN YOUR LEGS INTO A BUTTERFLY POSITION WHILE KEEPING YOUR UPPER BODY LIFTED AND ENGAGING YOUR CORE.
4. STRAIGHTEN ONE LEG TOWARDS THE CEILING WHILE KEEPING THE OTHER IN THE BUTTERFLY POSITION, ENGAGING YOUR CORE AND MAINTAINING STABILITY.
5. INHALE AS YOU LOWER YOUR UPPER BODY AND LEGS BACK DOWN TO THE MAT WITH CONTROL.

BENEFITS: HELPS INTEGRATE CORE STRENGTHENING WITH HIP MOBILITY EXERCISES, ENHANCING FLEXIBILITY, ABDOMINAL STRENGTH, AND OVERALL BODY COORDINATION FOR A COMPREHENSIVE PILATES WORKOUT.

"YOU CAN BE SO PROUD OF YOURSELF."

23. FROG CRUNCHES TO RAINBOWS – SUPERSET

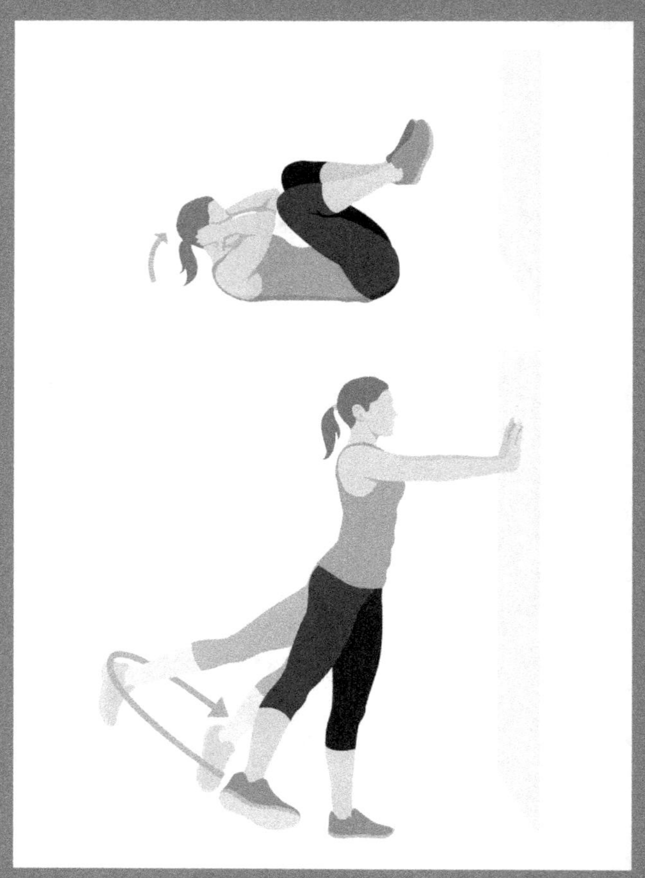

1. BEGIN LYING ON YOUR BACK WITH YOUR FEET FLAT AGAINST A WALL, KNEES BENT, AND ARMS BY YOUR SIDES.
2. EXHALE AS YOU LIFT YOUR HEAD, NECK, AND SHOULDERS OFF THE MAT, BRINGING YOUR KNEES TOWARDS YOUR CHEST WHILE REACHING YOUR HANDS TOWARDS YOUR ANKLES.
3. FROM THE CRUNCH POSITION, OPEN YOUR ARMS AND LEGS OUTWARDS, THEN EXHALE AS YOU BRING YOUR ARMS AND LEGS BACK TOGETHER, TRACING A RAINBOW MOTION WITH YOUR LIMBS.
4. INHALE AS YOU LOWER YOUR UPPER BODY AND LEGS BACK DOWN TO THE MAT WITH CONTROL.

BENEFITS: HELPS COMBINE CORE STRENGTHENING WITH DYNAMIC MOBILITY EXERCISES, PROMOTING ABDOMINAL TONING, FLEXIBILITY, AND OVERALL BODY COORDINATION FOR A BALANCED PILATES ROUTINE.

" YOU MADE IT. YOU ARE A ROCKSTAR."

24. FIRE HYDRANT TO BUTT PULSE   10 X

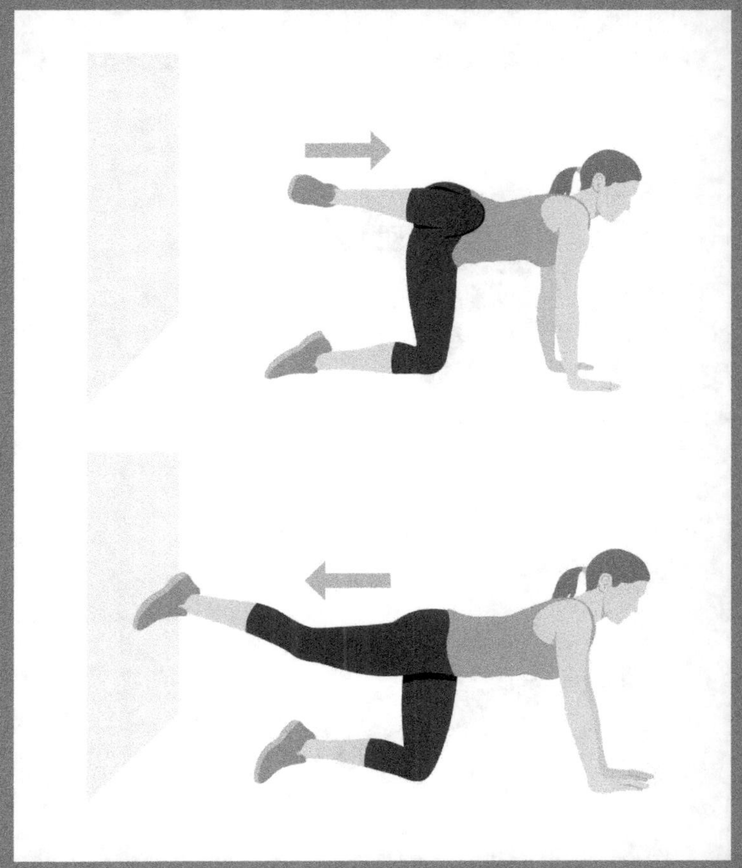

1. POSITIONING YOURSELF ON ALL FOURS WITH YOUR HANDS DIRECTLY UNDER YOUR SHOULDERS AND YOUR KNEES UNDER YOUR HIPS.
2. ENGAGE YOUR CORE MUSCLES TO MAINTAIN STABILITY THROUGHOUT THE MOVEMENT.
3. LIFT ONE LEG OUT TO THE SIDE, SIMILAR TO A DOG LIFTING ITS LEG AT A FIRE HYDRANT.
4. KEEP YOUR KNEE BENT AT A 90-DEGREE ANGLE AS YOU LIFT, MAINTAINING A STABLE PELVIS AND AVOIDING ANY ROTATION IN YOUR HIPS OR TORSO.
5. ONCE YOUR LEG IS LIFTED TO THE SIDE, PERFORM A CONTROLLED PULSE UPWARD WITH YOUR GLUTES. FOCUS ON SQUEEZING THE MUSCLES AT THE SIDE OF YOUR HIP TO LIFT YOUR LEG SLIGHTLY HIGHER WHILE KEEPING YOUR CORE ENGAGED TO STABILIZE YOUR BODY.
6. AFTER COMPLETING SEVERAL PULSES, SLOWLY LOWER YOUR LEG BACK DOWN TO THE STARTING POSITION.

BENEFITS: HELPS TONE AND STRENGTHEN THE BUTTOCKS WHILE ALSO IMPROVING HIP MOBILITY AND STABILITY.

'YOUR BODY NEEDS YOUR WORDS"

28 DAY CHALLENGE:

25.   HALF MOON LEG LIFT   10 X

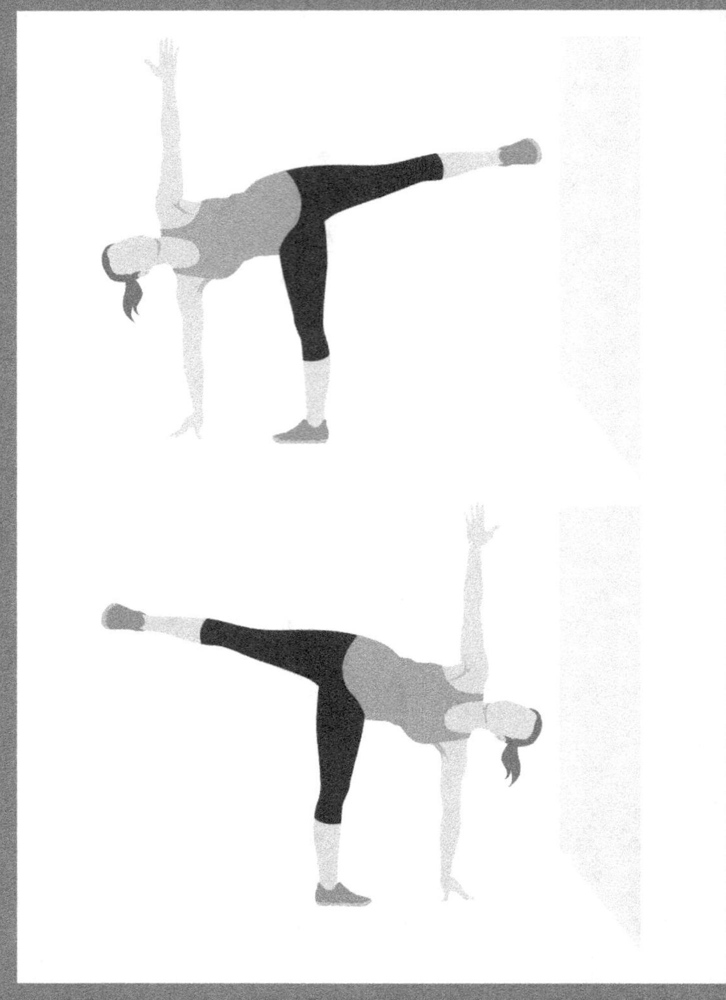

1. STAND SIDEWAYS TO A WALL FOR SUPPORT. WITH ONE HAND LIGHTLY TOUCHING THE FLOOR FOR BALANCE,
2. LIFT ONE LEG SIDEWAYS, KEEPING IT STRAIGHT AND PARALLEL TO THE FLOOR, WHILE ENGAGING THE OUTER THIGH AND GLUTE MUSCLES.
3. HOLD FOR A MOMENT AT THE TOP, THEN LOWER THE LEG WITH CONTROL.

BENEFITS: HELPS IMPROVE HIP STABILITY, STRENGTHENS THE LEG MUSCLES, AND ENHANCES OVERALL LOWER BODY STRENGTH AND TONE.

'BREATHE AND RELAX THROUGH YOUR WHOLE BODY "

COOL DOWN :

1. SPINE TWIST RIGHT AND LEFT　　10 X EACH SIDE

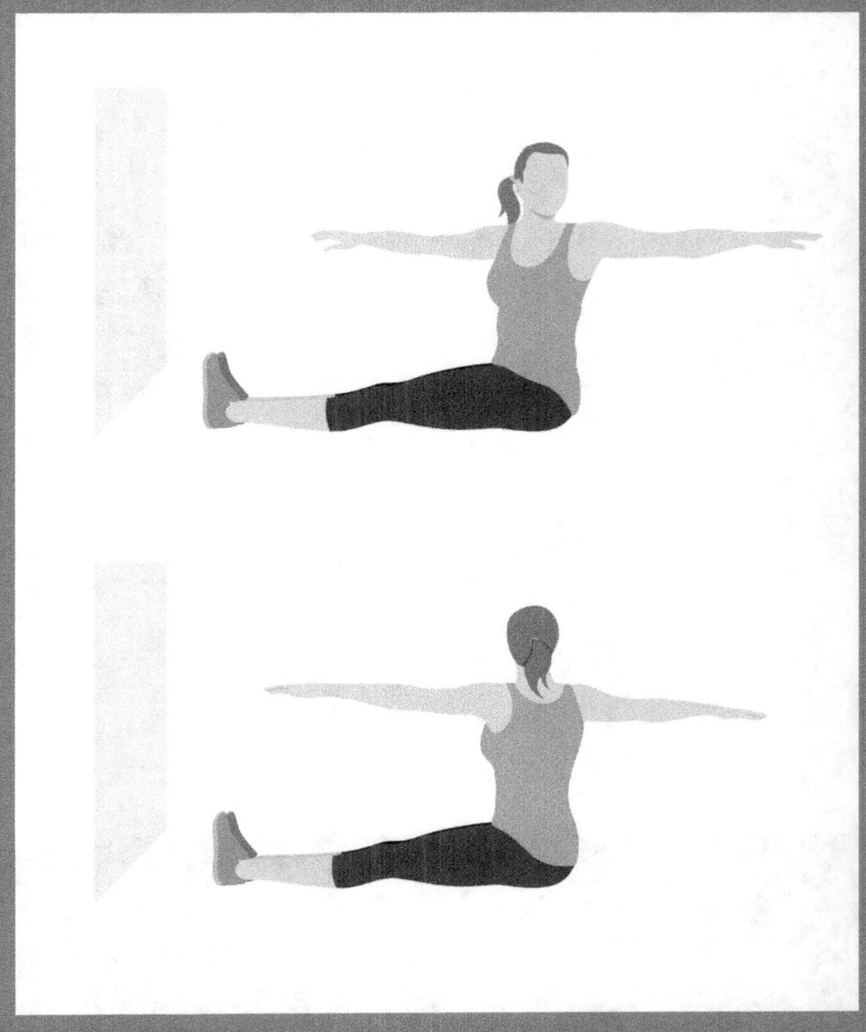

1. SIT TALL WITH LEGS EXTENDED. ARMS OUT TO THE SIDES AT SHOULDER HEIGHT.
2. TIGHTEN YOUR ABS.
3. EXHALE, TWIST TORSO TO THE RIGHT, KEEPING HIPS GROUNDED.
4. HOLD BRIEFLY, THEN INHALE BACK TO CENTER.
5. EXHALE, TWIST TORSO TO THE LEFT.
6. HOLD BRIEFLY, THEN INHALE BACK TO CENTER.
7. ALTERNATE TWISTS

BENEFITS: HELPS IMPROVE SPINAL MOBILITY AND CORE STRENGTH

'SEE YOUR BODY WITH YOUR BEST LENSES.'

COOL DOWN :

2. NECK ROTATION   10 X EACH SIDE

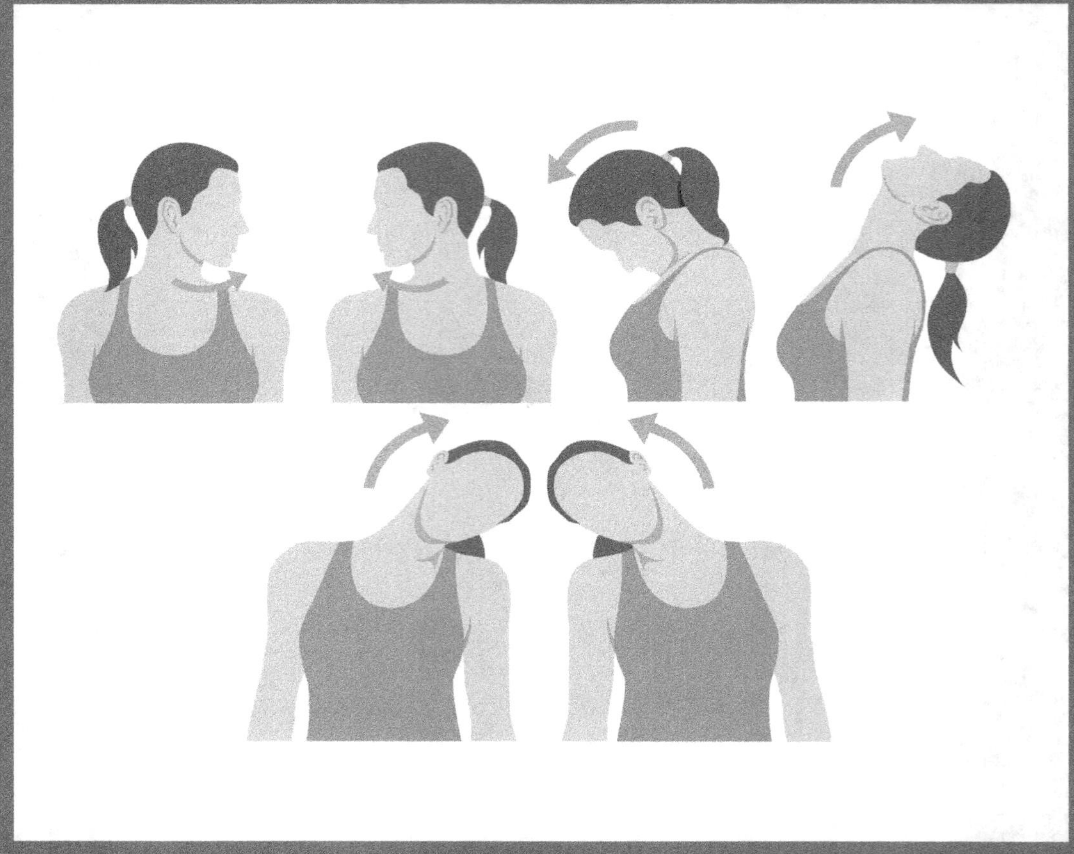

1. SIT OR STAND TALL WITH YOUR SHOULDERS RELAXED AND YOUR SPINE STRAIGHT.
2. KEEP YOUR ABDOMINAL MUSCLES GENTLY ENGAGED TO SUPPORT YOUR SPINE.
3. SLOWLY TURN YOUR HEAD TO THE RIGHT, KEEPING YOUR CHIN PARALLEL TO THE GROUND. ONLY ROTATE AS FAR AS COMFORTABLE.
4. HOLD THE POSITION BRIEFLY, FEELING A GENTLE STRETCH. THEN, RETURN YOUR HEAD TO THE CENTER.
5. REPEAT THE ROTATION TO THE LEFT SIDE, AGAIN HOLDING BRIEFLY BEFORE RETURNING TO CENTER.
6. EXHALE AS YOU TUCK YOUR CHIN TOWARD YOUR CHEST, BRINGING YOUR HEAD DOWN. KEEP YOUR SHOULDERS RELAXED.
7. HOLD THE POSITION BRIEFLY, FEELING A STRETCH IN THE BACK OF YOUR NECK. THEN, INHALE AS YOU RETURN YOUR HEAD TO THE NEUTRAL POSITION.

BENEFITS: HELPS IMPROVE NECK FLEXIBILITY AND RELIEVES TENSION IN THE NECK MUSCLES.

'PEACE IS COMING ALL OVER YOUR BODY.'

COOL DOWN :

3. SIDE TO SIDE STRETCH   10 X EACH SIDE

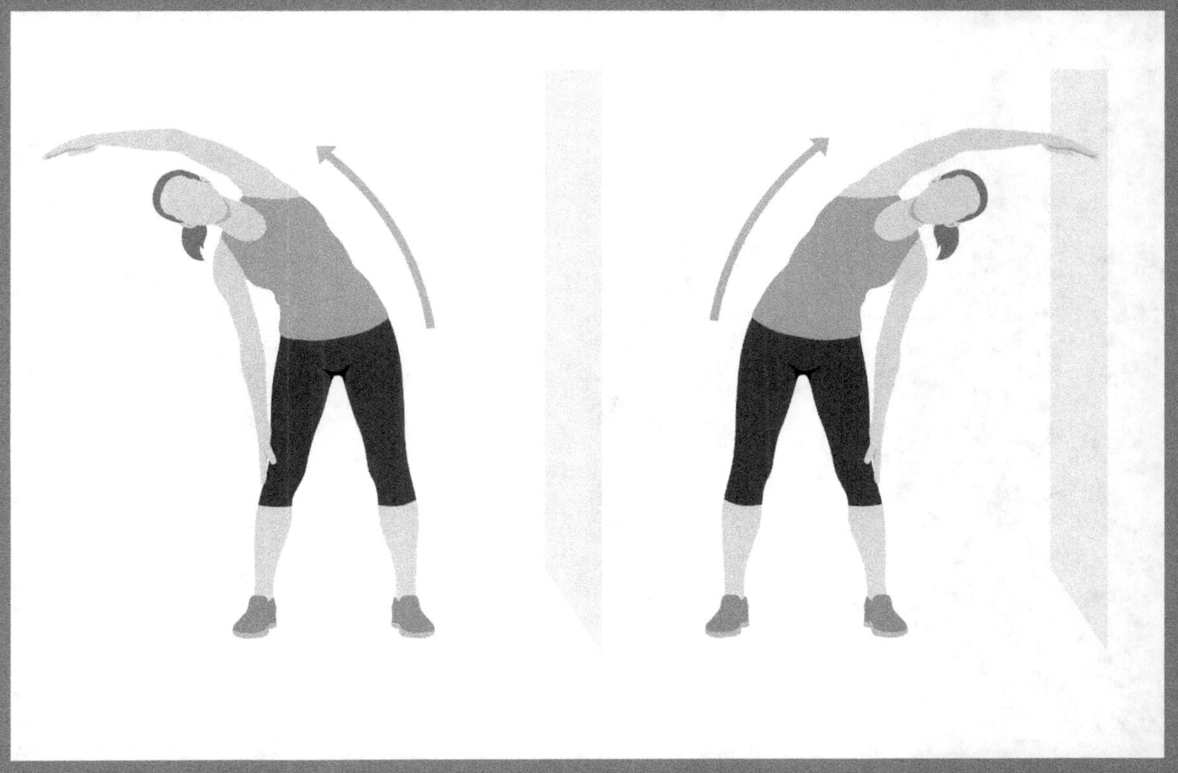

1. SIT OR STAND TALL WITH YOUR SHOULDERS RELAXED AND YOUR SPINE STRAIGHT.
2. INHALE AS YOU REACH ONE ARM UP OVERHEAD, KEEPING IT STRAIGHT AND CLOSE TO YOUR EAR.
3. EXHALE AS YOU GENTLY LEAN YOUR TORSO TO THE OPPOSITE SIDE, FEELING A STRETCH ALONG THE ENTIRE SIDE OF YOUR BODY, FROM YOUR FINGERTIPS DOWN TO YOUR HIP.
4. HOLD THE STRETCH FOR A FEW SECONDS, FEELING A GENTLE ELONGATION THROUGH YOUR SIDE BODY.
5. INHALE AS YOU SLOWLY RETURN TO THE UPRIGHT POSITION, BRINGING YOUR ARM BACK DOWN TO YOUR SIDE.
6. INHALE TO RAISE THE OPPOSITE ARM OVERHEAD, THEN EXHALE AS YOU LEAN TO THE OPPOSITE SIDE, FEELING THE STRETCH ALONG THE OTHER SIDE OF YOUR BODY.
7. HOLD THE STRETCH BRIEFLY, THEN INHALE TO RETURN TO THE CENTER POSITION.

BENEFITS: HELPS STRETCH THE MUSCLES ALONG THE SIDES OF YOUR BODY, INCLUDING THE LATS, OBLIQUES, AND INTERCOSTAL MUSCLES, WHILE ALSO PROMOTING SPINAL MOBILITY AND POSTURE.

'HAVE THE BEST INTENTIONS TO YOURSELF."

COOL DOWN :

4. WALL CHEST OPENER   10 X EACH SIDE

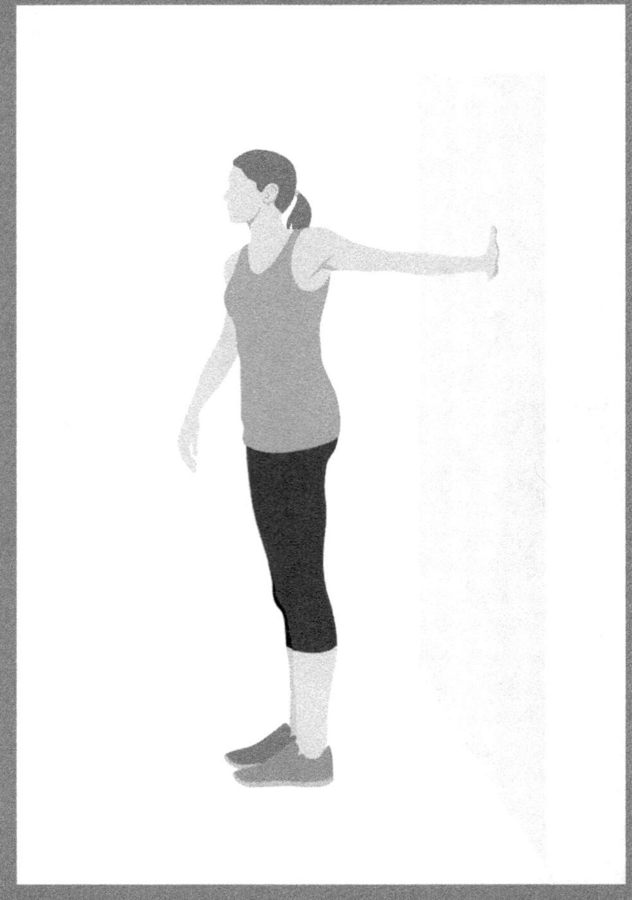

1. STAND FACING A WALL WITH YOUR FEET HIP-WIDTH APART.
2. PLACE HAND ON WALL: EXTEND ONE ARM OUT TO THE SIDE AT SHOULDER HEIGHT, PALM FLAT AGAINST THE WALL, FINGERS POINTING BACKWARD.
3. OPEN CHEST: SLOWLY ROTATE YOUR BODY AWAY FROM THE WALL, KEEPING YOUR ARM EXTENDED AND YOUR HAND IN CONTACT WITH THE WALL. YOU SHOULD FEEL A STRETCH ACROSS THE FRONT OF YOUR CHEST AND SHOULDER.
4. HOLD AND FEEL THE STRETCH: HOLD THE STRETCH FOR A FEW SECONDS, FOCUSING ON OPENING UP THROUGH THE CHEST WHILE KEEPING YOUR SHOULDERS RELAXED.
5. RETURN TO STARTING POSITION: SLOWLY ROTATE YOUR BODY BACK TO THE STARTING POSITION, BRINGING YOUR ARM BACK TO YOUR SIDE.
6. REPEAT ON THE OTHER SIDE: EXTEND YOUR OPPOSITE ARM OUT TO THE SIDE, PALM FLAT AGAINST THE WALL, AND REPEAT THE STRETCH ON THE OTHER SIDE.

BENEFITS: HELPS TO STRETCH THE CHEST MUSCLES, IMPROVE SHOULDER MOBILITY, AND COUNTERACT THE EFFECTS OF HUNCHING OR ROUNDED SHOULDERS.

'SAY THREE THINGS YOU LIKE ABOUT YOUR BODY."

COOL DOWN :

5. WALL SUPPORTED FORWARD FOLD   10 X

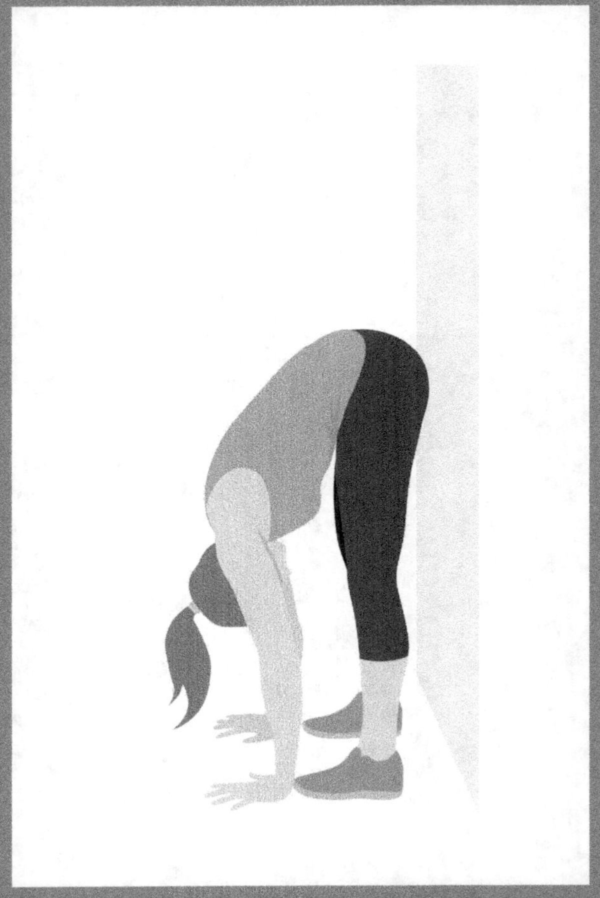

1. STAND FACING A WALL WITH YOUR FEET HIP-WIDTH APART.
2. REACH YOUR ARMS UP AND PRESS YOUR PALMS AGAINST THE WALL, SHOULDER-WIDTH APART, AT ABOUT CHEST HEIGHT.
3. SLOWLY HINGE FORWARD AT YOUR HIPS, KEEPING YOUR ARMS EXTENDED AND YOUR PALMS PRESSING INTO THE WALL.
4. AS YOU FOLD FORWARD, FOCUS ON LENGTHENING YOUR SPINE AND REACHING YOUR TAILBONE TOWARD THE WALL BEHIND YOU.
5. ALLOW YOUR HEAD AND NECK TO RELAX, LETTING THEM HANG NATURALLY.
6. YOU SHOULD FEEL A GENTLE STRETCH ALONG YOUR SPINE, HAMSTRINGS, AND SHOULDERS.
7. HOLD THE STRETCH FOR A FEW DEEP BREATHS, ALLOWING YOUR BODY TO RELAX INTO THE POSITION.
8. TO COME OUT OF THE STRETCH, SLOWLY ROLL BACK UP TO STANDING, STACKING EACH VERTEBRA OF YOUR SPINE ONE AT A TIME.

BENEFITS: HELPS TO RELEASE TENSION IN THE BACK, HAMSTRINGS, AND SHOULDERS, WHILE ALSO PROMOTING FLEXIBILITY AND SPINAL MOBILITY.

"BE ONE WITH YOUR BODY."

15 MINUTES WORKOUT:

OPTION 1:

HERE ARE THREE 15-MINUTE WORKOUT OPTIONS UTILIZING WARM-UP, COOL-DOWN, AND WORKOUT EXERCISES. EACH WORKOUT TARGETS MULTIPLE MUSCLE GROUPS, PROVIDING A HOLISTIC EXERCISE EXPERIENCE. CHOOSE ONE WARM-UP AND ONE COOL-DOWN EXERCISE, ALONG WITH FOUR WORKOUT EXERCISES FROM THE PROVIDED LIST TO CREATE A WELL-ROUNDED ROUTINE

EXERCISE (10 MINUTES): PERFORM THE FOLLOWING EXERCISES IN CIRCUIT FASHION WITH MINIMAL REST BETWEEN EACH:

WARM UP:	
PERFORM DYNAMIC STRETCHES SUCH AS ARM CIRCLES, LEG SWINGS, AND TORSO ROTATIONS TO PREPARE YOUR BODY.	PAGE 17-21

WORKOUT:	
WALL SQUATS: 4 SETS OF 10 REPS	PAGE 22
SIDE PLANK HIP OPENER - RIGHT/LEFT: HOLD FOR 30 SECONDS, THEN 10 HIP OPENERS ON EACH SIDE	PAGE 29
WALL PIKE PRESS: 4 SETS OF 10 REPS	PAGE 38
FROG CRUNCHES TO RAINBOWS SUPERSET: 4 SETS OF 12 REPS FOR EACH EXERCISE	PAGE 44

COOL DOWN:	
SPINE TWIST RIGHT AND LEFT	PAGE 47
WALL CHEST OPENER: HOLD FOR 30 SECONDS EACH SIDE	PAGE 50

15 MINUTES WORKOUT:

OPTION 2:

EXERCISE (10 MINUTES): PERFORM THE FOLLOWING EXERCISES IN CIRCUIT FASHION WITH MINIMAL REST BETWEEN EACH:

WARM UP:	
START WITH LIGHT CARDIO, SUCH AS MARCHING IN PLACE OR GENTLE JUMPING JACKS, TO INCREASE HEART RATE AND WARM UP MUSCLES.	DO IT FOR 5 MIN.

WORKOUT:	
WALL PUSH-UPS: 4 SETS OF 12 REPS	PAGE 25
SIDE PLANK HIP OPENER - RIGHT/LEFT: HOLD FOR 1MINUTE THEN PERFORM 10 HIP OPENERS ON EACH SIDE	PAGE 29
WALL BRIDGE WITH ALTERNATING LEG EXTENSIONS: 4 SETS OF 12 REPS	PAGE 37
FIRE HYDRANT TO BUTT PULSE : 4 SETS OF 10 REPS FORWARD AND BACKWARD	PAGE 45

COOL DOWN	
SIDE TO SIDE STRETCH	PAGE 49
WALL SUPPORTED FORWARD FOLD	PAGE 51

15 MINUTES WORKOUT:

OPTION 3:

EXERCISE (10 MINUTES): PERFORM THE FOLLOWING EXERCISES IN CIRCUIT FASHION WITH MINIMAL REST BETWEEN EACH:

WARM UP:	
WALL ROLL DOWN: 1 MINUTE	PAGE 20
HIP ROTATION: 1 MINUTE EACH SIDE	PAGE 19

WORKOUT:	
TOE TAP CRUNCH: 4 SETS OF 12 REPS	PAGE 26
WALL BRIDGE WITH MARCHING: 4 SETS OF 12 REPS	PAGE 33
EXPLOSIVE WALL PUSH-UPS: 4 SETS OF 10 REPS	PAGE 35
WALL PUSH-UPS TO SIDE PLANK HIP OPENER SUPERSET: 4 SETS OF 10 REPS FOR EACH EXERCISE	PAGE 42

COOL DOWN	
WALL CHEST OPENER: HOLD FOR 15 SECONDS ON EACH SIDE.	PAGE 50
ALL SUPPORTED FORWARD FOLD: HOLD FOR 15 SECONDS ON EACH SIDE.	PAGE 51

BONUS 1

YOU KNOW, IT'S FUNNY HOW SOMETHING AS SIMPLE AS BREATHING CAN HOLD SO MUCH POWER, YET WE OFTEN OVERLOOK ITS SIGNIFICANCE.

OUR BREATH IS OUR LIFE FORCE – IT'S WHAT BRINGS US INTO THIS WORLD AND KEEPS US GOING EVERY DAY. BUT IT'S MORE THAN JUST A BIOLOGICAL FUNCTION; IT'S A TOOL FOR TRANSFORMATION.

WHEN WE TAKE THE TIME TO TUNE INTO OUR BREATH, TO REALLY CONNECT WITH IT, WE UNLOCK A WHOLE NEW LEVEL OF POTENTIAL – NOT JUST IN OUR WORKOUTS, BUT IN OUR ENTIRE BEING.

IT'S INCREDIBLE HOW SOMETHING AS BASIC AS BREATHING DEEPLY AND INTENTIONALLY CAN HAVE SUCH PROFOUND EFFECTS ON OUR HEALTH AND WELL-BEING.

AND THE BEST PART? YOU DON'T NEED FANCY EQUIPMENT OR EXPENSIVE GEAR TO TAP INTO THIS POWER.

ALL YOU NEED IS YOURSELF AND A LITTLE BIT OF SPACE – MAYBE EVEN JUST A WALL TO LEAN ON FOR SUPPORT.

SO LET'S TAKE A MOMENT TO HONOR THE BREATH, TO APPRECIATE ITS INCREDIBLE POTENCY,
AND TO HARNESS ITS ENERGY TO FUEL OUR JOURNEY TOWARDS A STRONGER, HEALTHIER SELF.

BONUS 1

DIAPHRAGMATIC BREATHING (BELLY BREATHING):

FIND A COMFORTABLE SEATED POSITION OR LIE DOWN ON YOUR BACK WITH KNEES BENT AND FEET FLAT ON THE FLOOR.

- PLACE ONE HAND ON YOUR CHEST AND THE OTHER ON YOUR ABDOMEN.
- INHALE DEEPLY THROUGH YOUR NOSE, ALLOWING YOUR BELLY TO RISE AS YOU FILL YOUR LUNGS WITH AIR. FOCUS ON EXPANDING YOUR ABDOMEN RATHER THAN LIFTING YOUR CHEST.
- EXHALE SLOWLY THROUGH YOUR MOUTH, DRAWING YOUR NAVEL IN TOWARDS YOUR SPINE TO FULLY EMPTY YOUR LUNGS.
- REPEAT THIS DEEP BELLY BREATHING FOR SEVERAL CYCLES, AIMING FOR A SLOW AND STEADY RHYTHM.
-
- DECREASE THE WORK OF BREATHING BY SLOWING YOUR BREATHING RATE.

THIS TECHNIQUE HELPS WITH REDUCING THE BLOOD PRESSURE, HEART RATE AND IMPROVES RELAXATION.
IT IMPROVES MUSCLE FUNCTION DURING EXERCISES AND PREVENTS STRAIN.

IT MAKES IT EASIER FOR YOUR BODY TO RELEASE GAS WASTE FROM YOUR LUNGS. IT'S GREAT FOR ASTHMA, STRESS AND ANXIETY.

BONUS 1

4-7-8 BREATHING TECHNIQUE:

- SIT OR LIE DOWN IN A COMFORTABLE POSITION, WITH YOUR BACK STRAIGHT AND SHOULDERS RELAXED.
- CLOSE YOUR EYES AND TAKE A DEEP BREATH IN THROUGH YOUR NOSE FOR A COUNT OF 4 SECONDS.
- HOLD YOUR BREATH FOR A COUNT OF 7 SECONDS.
- EXHALE SLOWLY AND COMPLETELY THROUGH YOUR MOUTH FOR A COUNT OF 8 SECONDS, MAKING A WHOOSHING SOUND AS YOU RELEASE THE AIR.
- REPEAT THIS CYCLE SEVERAL TIMES, FOCUSING ON THE SMOOTH AND EVEN FLOW OF YOUR BREATH.

IT HELPS YOUR OVERALL HEALTH. IT CAN HELP YOU TO FALL ASLEEP AND STAY ASLEEP AND REDUCES STRESS.

IT MANAGES CRAVING AS WELL AND SPUR OF ANGER. IMPROVE HEART AND BLOOD FUNCTION AND REDUCES BLOOD PRESSURE.

BONUS 1

BOX BREATHING:

- SIT OR STAND COMFORTABLY WITH YOUR SPINE STRAIGHT AND SHOULDERS RELAXED.
- INHALE DEEPLY THROUGH YOUR NOSE FOR A COUNT OF 4 SECONDS, FILLING YOUR LUNGS WITH AIR.
- HOLD YOUR BREATH AT THE TOP OF THE INHALATION FOR A COUNT OF 4 SECONDS.
- EXHALE SLOWLY AND COMPLETELY THROUGH YOUR MOUTH FOR A COUNT OF 4 SECONDS, EMPTYING YOUR LUNGS.
- HOLD YOUR BREATH AT THE BOTTOM OF THE EXHALATION FOR A COUNT OF 4 SECONDS.
- REPEAT THIS BOX BREATHING PATTERN FOR SEVERAL CYCLES, FOCUSING ON THE EQUAL LENGTH OF EACH INHALE, HOLD, EXHALE, AND HOLD.

THIS TECHNIQUE HELPS WITH TO CONTROL HYPERVENTILATION AS YOU CAN INSTRUCT YOUR LUNGS TO BREATHE RHYTHMICALLY BUT ALSO IT HELPS TO REFOCUS WHEN YOU ARE HAVING A BUSY OR STRESSFUL DAY. IT HELPS TO SLEEP BETTER AND REDUCES ANXIETY AND STRESS.

THESE BREATHING EXERCISES CAN HELP CALM YOUR MIND, REDUCE STRESS, AND PREPARE YOUR BODY FOR PHYSICAL ACTIVITY BY INCREASING OXYGEN FLOW AND PROMOTING RELAXATION.

EXPERIMENT WITH DIFFERENT TECHNIQUES TO FIND WHAT WORKS BEST FOR YOU, AND INCORPORATE THEM INTO YOUR PRE-WORKOUT ROUTINE FOR OPTIMAL RESULTS.

BONUS 2

IF YOU'RE LOOKING TO KICK YOUR WORKOUT UP A NOTCH AND TAKE A MORE HOLISTIC APPROACH TO YOUR FITNESS ROUTINE, LET ME INTRODUCE YOU TO SOMETHING PRETTY INCREDIBLE – COLD PLUNGES. PICTURE THIS: A QUICK DIP INTO AN ICY BATH OR STARTING WITH COLD SHOWERS.

NOW, I KNOW IT SOUNDS INTENSE, BUT HEAR ME OUT. COLD PLUNGES DO WONDERS FOR YOUR BODY. THEY BOOST YOUR IMMUNITY, REGULATE BLOOD PRESSURE, AND EVEN HELP WITH WEIGHT LOSS.

PLUS, THEY'RE A GAME-CHANGER FOR EASING SORE MUSCLES AND MIGHT JUST GIVE YOU THE BEST NIGHT'S SLEEP OF YOUR LIFE. NOT TO MENTION, THEY'RE FANTASTIC FOR REDUCING INFLAMMATION AND SHARPENING YOUR FOCUS.

OF COURSE, LIKE ANYTHING NEW, IT'S IMPORTANT TO DO YOUR RESEARCH AND MAKE SURE IT'S THE RIGHT FIT FOR YOU BEFORE DIVING IN – PUN INTENDED.

SO, IF YOU'RE CURIOUS ABOUT COLD PLUNGES, TAKE THE TIME TO GATHER ALL THE INFO YOU NEED AND SEE IF IT ALIGNS WITH YOUR HEALTH AND FITNESS GOALS.

TRUST ME, IT'S WORTH EXPLORING!

BONUS 3

MEDITATION OFFERS VARIOUS APPROACHES THESE DAYS. SIMPLY PUT, IT'S ABOUT DEEP CONTEMPLATION, A PROCESS THAT TRANSFORMS THE MIND THROUGH WHAT WE FOCUS ON.

WHAT WE CHOOSE TO CONTEMPLATE MATTERS GREATLY BECAUSE IT SHAPES WHO WE BECOME. OUR THOUGHTS INFLUENCE OUR REALITY, SO IT'S CRUCIAL TO BE MINDFUL OF WHAT WE FOCUS ON.

WHEN WE RECOGNIZE SOMETHING GREATER THAN OURSELVES, IT BRINGS CLARITY AND FOCUS, REMINDING US OF OUR IDENTITY AND POTENTIAL TRANSFORMATION.

BY PRACTICING STILLNESS AND AWARENESS OF OUR SURROUNDINGS WHILE FOCUSING ON SOMETHING LARGER THAN OURSELVES, WE OPEN OURSELVES TO NEW INSIGHTS AND EXPERIENCES.

THIS JOURNEY HELPS US ALIGN WITH OUR DESIRES AND FEEL A SENSE OF PEACE AND LOVE WITHIN.

INCORPORATING MEDITATION INTO YOUR WALL PILATES ROUTINE CAN ENHANCE YOUR OVERALL WELL-BEING. IT'S SCIENTIFICALLY PROVEN TO REDUCE STRESS, ANXIETY, AND PROMOTE EMOTIONAL HEALTH.

IT ALSO BOOSTS SELF-AWARENESS, AIDS IN BETTER SLEEP, LOWERS BLOOD PRESSURE, AND HELPS MANAGE PAIN.

IT'S A POWERFUL TOOL THAT COMPLEMENTS PHYSICAL EXERCISE, LEAVING YOU FEELING EVEN MORE PEACEFUL AND PREPARED FOR WHATEVER THE DAY BRINGS.

BONUS 3

I'VE GOT A MEDITATION THAT YOU MIGHT LOVE AS WELL.
IT WORKS FOR ME AND I AM ALMOST SURE THAT IT MIGHT WORK FOR YOU.

FIRST, PICTURE YOURSELF IN YOUR FAVORITE PLACE, WHETHER IT'S REAL OR IMAGINARY.
MAYBE IT'S A COZY BEACH, A PEACEFUL FOREST, OR EVEN THE MAGICAL WORLD OF NARNIA.

ONCE YOU'RE THERE, TAKE SOME DEEP BREATHS AND RELAX. USE THE TECHNIQUES MENTIONED PREVIOUSLY.

THEN, IMAGINE SOMEONE SPECIAL JOINING YOU – SOMEONE WHO KNOWS YOU INSIDE AND OUT, ALMOST LIKE THEY'VE BEEN WITH YOU SINCE THE BEGINNING.
YOU MIGHT NOT KNOW HIM BUT THAT'S OKAY. HE HAS THE BEST INTENTION FOR YOU.
THIS PERSON IS GOING TO GIVE YOU A GIFT. TRY TO PICTURE WHAT IT MIGHT BE.

THEY MIGHT EVEN ASK SOMETHING OF YOU IN RETURN – IT'S UP TO YOU! YOU DON'T HAVE TO.
AFTER THE EXCHANGE, HE'LL WHISPER SOMETHING TO YOU. LISTEN CLOSELY AND FEEL HOW IT TOUCHES YOUR HEART AND YOUR SPIRIT.
THEN, HE WILL LEAVE. IT'S ALL GOOD.

IT'S ALWAYS SOMETHING POSITIVE AND UPLIFTING, SO LET IT SINK IN.
TAKE A MOMENT TO REST AND BREATHE DEEPLY, FEELING YOUR BODY RELAX IN THAT SPACE.

WHEN YOU'RE READY, OPEN YOUR EYES AND APPRECIATE THE CALMNESS YOU'VE FOUND. YOU CAN CARRY THIS FEELING WITH YOU WHEREVER YOU GO – IT REALLY DOES WONDERS!

BONUS 4

WHILE WALL PILATES PRIMARILY FOCUSES ON STRENGTH, FLEXIBILITY, AND STABILITY,

THERE ARE SEVERAL EXERCISES THAT CAN INDIRECTLY SUPPORT WEIGHT LOSS GOALS BY ENGAGING MULTIPLE MUSCLE GROUPS AND INCREASING CALORIE BURN. FOCUS ON THOSE ONES OR INCORPORATE THOSE IN YOUR ROUTINE.

HERE ARE SOME EXAMPLES:

- WALL SQUATS TO BUTTERFLY CRUNCH: PAGE 39 – 4 SETS OF 10 REPS

- WALL PUSH-UPS: PAGE 25 – 4 SETS OF 10 REPS

- WALL PLANK WITH KNEE DRIVES: PAGE 36 – 4 SETS OF 10 REPS

- WALL BRIDGE WITH MARCHING: PAGE 33 – 4 SETS OF 10 REPS

- WALL SIDE PLANK HIP OPENER: PAGE 29 – 4 SETS OF 10 REPS

BONUS 5

YOU GOT THIS!!!

TRACK YOUR PROGRESS FOR AT LEAST 3 MONTHS AND WITNESS YOUR INCREDIBLE RESULTS.

IN JUST A MONTH, YOU CAN TRANSFORM INTO A NEW AND EMPOWERED VERSION OF YOURSELF.
REMEMBER, YOU'RE A ROCKSTAR!

KEEP YOURSELF MOTIVATED BY FILLING IN THESE SPACES.

YOU'LL BE AMAZED AT HOW FAR YOU'VE COME.

YOU GOT THIS!!!

BE YOU!

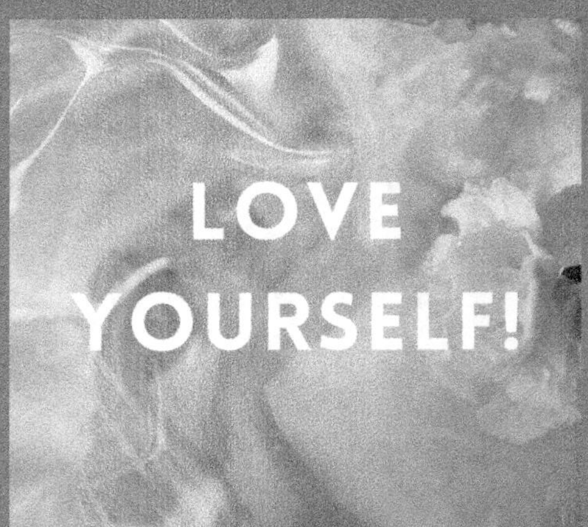

BEAUTY

28 DAYS CHALLENGE

CHECK THE CASE AS SOON AS YOU WERE ABLE TO DO IT.

MONTH OF:

1	2	3	4	5
6	7	8	9	10
11	12	13	14	15
16	17	18	19	20
21	22	23	24	25
26	27	28	29	30

28 DAYS CHALLENGE

CHECK THE CASE AS SOON AS YOU WERE ABLE TO DO IT.

MONTH OF:

1	2	3	4	5
6	7	8	9	10
11	12	13	14	15
16	17	18	19	20
21	22	23	24	25
26	27	28	29	30

28 DAYS CHALLENGE

CHECK THE CASE AS SOON AS YOU WERE ABLE TO DO IT.

MONTH OF:

1	2	3	4	5
6	7	8	9	10
11	12	13	14	15
16	17	18	19	20
21	22	23	24	25
26	27	28	29	30

28 DAYS CHALLENGE

CHECK THE CASE AS SOON AS YOU WERE ABLE TO DO IT.

MONTH OF:

1	2	3	4	5
6	7	8	9	10
11	12	13	14	15
16	17	18	19	20
21	22	23	24	25
26	27	28	29	30

WHAT A HERO! YOU DID IT:

KEEP THE GOOD WORK!

THANK YOU FOR CHOOSING THIS INCREDIBLE WALL PILATES BOOK, DESIGNED TO KNOW YOURSELF BETTER AND TO UNLOCK YOUR FULL POTENTIAL.

YOUR SUPPORT MEANS THE WORLD TO ME, AND I'M TRULY GRATEFUL FOR THE OPPORTUNITY TO SHARE THIS WORKOUT JOURNEY WITH YOU.

IF YOU'VE ENJOYED IMMERSING YOURSELF IN THESE WORKOUT PAGES AND FOUND THEM TO BE A SOURCE OF EMPOWERMENT AND TRANSFORMATION.

I WOULD BE IMMENSELY GRATEFUL IF YOU COULD TAKE A MOMENT TO LEAVE A REVIEW ON AMAZON.

YOUR FEEDBACK WILL HELP OTHERS DISCOVER THE NEED AND EMPOWERMENT THIS BOOK HAS TO OFFER.

THANK YOU FOR YOUR KIND WORDS AND FOR BEING A PART OF THIS BEAUTIFUL JOURNEY TOGETHER.

IF YOU WANT TO GET IT ON YOUR PHONE. SEND AN EMAIL TO INFO@OFLOWLY.COM TO GET THE PASSWORD.

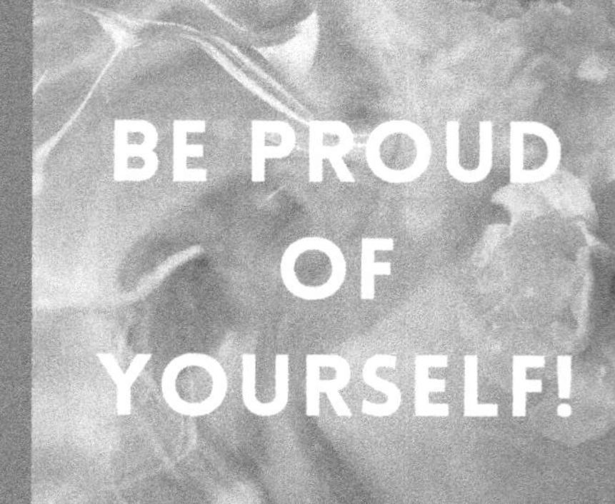

BE PROUD OF YOURSELF!

IMPORTANT!